Study Guide to Accompany

NURSING FUNDAMENTALS:

CARING & CLINICAL DECISION MAKING

RICK DANIELS

Questions Prepared by

Vicky P. Kent, PhD, RN
Assistant Professor
Community Health Nursing
Towson University
Towson, Maryland

Kim McCarron, MS, RN
Clinical Assistant Professor
Medical Surgical Nursing
Nursing Skills Lab Coordinator
Towson University
Towson, Maryland

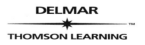

DELMAR
™
THOMSON LEARNING

Australia Canada Mexico Singapore Spain United Kingdom United States

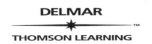

Study Guide to Accompany
Nursing Fundamentals: Caring & Clinical Decision Making
by Rick Daniels
prepared by Vicky P. Kent and Kim McCarron

Vice President, Health Care Business Unit:
William Brottmiller

Editorial Director:
Cathy L. Esperti

Acquisitions Editor:
Matthew Filimonov

Senior Developmental Editors:
Marah Bellegarde, Elisabeth F. Williams

Editorial Assistant:
Patricia Osborn

Marketing Director:
Jennifer McAvey

Marketing Channel Manager:
Tamara Caruso

Marketing Coordinator:
Karen Summerlin

Production Manager:
Barbara A. Bullock

Project Editor:
Mary Ellen Cox

Art/Design Specialist:
Connie Lundberg-Watkins

Production Coordinator:
Kenneth McGrath

Technology Director:
Laurie K. Davis

Technology Project Manager:
Victoria Moore

Technology Production Coordinator:
Sherry Conners

Library of Congress Cataloging-in-Publication Data

ISBN: 0766838374

INTERNATIONAL DIVISIONS LIST

Asia (including India):
Thomson Learning
60 Albert Street, #15-01
Albert Complex
Singapore 189969
Tel 65 336-6411
Fax 65 336-7411

Australia/New Zealand:
Nelson
102 Dodds Street
South Melbourne
Victoria 3205
Australia
Tel 61 (0)3 9685-4111
Fax 61 (0)3 9685-4111

Latin America:
Thomson Learning
Seneca 53
Colonia Polanco
11560 Mexico, D.F. Mexico
Tel (525) 281-2906
Fax (525) 281-2656

Canada:
Nelson
1120 Birchmount Road
Toronto, Ontario
Canada M1K 5G4
Tel (416) 752-9100
Fax (416) 752-8102

UK/Europe/Middle East/Africa:
Thomson Learning
Berkshire House
1680-173 High Holborn
London WC1V 7AA
United Kingdom
Tel 44 (0)20 497-1422
Fax 44 (0)20 497-1426

Spain (includes Portugal):
Paraninfo
Calle Megallanes 25
28015 Madrid
España
Tel 34 (0)91 446-3350
Fax 34 (0)91 445-6218

NOTICE TO THE READER

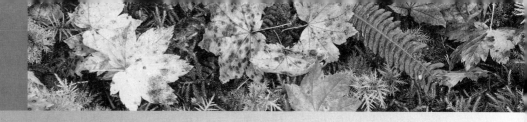

Contents

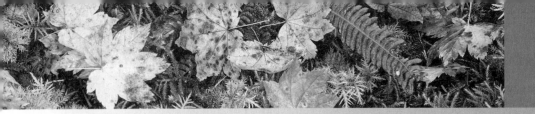

Preface

This study guide is designed to accompany Nursing Fundamentals: Caring & Clinical Decision Making, by Rick Daniels. Each of the 48 chapters in this guide was created to facilitate student learning and refine student skills. By using this guide at home and in the clinical setting, you will work with important concepts and begin to apply them to real-life situations.

The exercises in the workbook were developed from the content in the core text. For effective study, completing a chapter in the text is recommended prior to beginning the related chapter in the workbook.

A variety of review questions is provided based upon each chapter content. Types of questions include multiple choice, matching, true-false, and completion. There are also critical-thinking questions to help you hone your ability to problem solve. Answers to the questions appear at the end of the book.

CHAPTER 1

Evolution of Nursing Practice

1. Nurses focus primarily on a client's

    a. illness.

    b. response to illness.

    c. ability to pay for health care services.

    d. technological interventions and therapies.

2. In Western Europe, during the Middle Ages, nursing care was provided by

    a. priestesses.

    b. the Sisters of Mercy.

    c. orders of knights.

    d. Jesuit priests.

3. During the Crimean War, Florence Nightingale implemented nursing practices that contributed to a drop in mortality rate from 42.7% to 2.2%. What were these practices?

    a. The infected and wounded were placed in private quarters.

    b. The healing environment was improved by the addition of light and fresh air.

    c. Mortality rates among soldiers were statistically analyzed.

    d. Penicillin was introduced and used experimentally on soldiers with infected wounds.

4. Florence Nightingale revolutionized nursing by

    a. establishing the first hospital in Britain where nurses could practice without the direction of physicians.

    b. changing the image of nurses from handmaidens to professionals with autonomy.

    c. educating nurses in theoretical concepts as well as clinical skills.

    d. developing the first documentation system for client care.

5. Which of the following women in nursing history founded the Red Cross in the United States?

   a. Dorothea Dix

   b. Lillian Wald

   c. Annie Goodrich

   d. Clara Barton

6. Which of the following nursing leaders founded several nursing organizations and supported the rights of nursing students?

   a. Isabel Hampton Robb

   b. Adelaide Nutting

   c. Jane Delano

   d. Lavinia Dock

7. The American Nurses Association (ANA) was founded in

   a. 1900.

   b. 1911.

   c. 1912.

   d. 1921.

8. Match the decade in the left column with the event that occurred in that decade from the right column.

   _____ 1920s   a. Proliferation of HMOs

   _____ 1930s   b. Creation of Medicare and Medicaid

   _____ 1940s   c. The Brown Report

   _____ 1950s   d. Women can vote

   _____ 1960s   e. The advent of Blue Cross and Blue Shield

   _____ 1970s   f. The advent of LPN programs

   _____ 1980s   g. Health care reform

   _____ 1990s   h. Nurse practitioners reimbursed directly for their services

9. Which of the following nursing leaders established the Frontier Nursing Service, thereby introducing health care delivery to rural America?

    a. Mary Breckinridge

    b. Adelaide Nutting

    c. Clara Barton

    d. Lavinia Dock

10. Margaret Sanger, an early feminist nurse, is best known for her

    a. work with the women's suffrage movement.

    b. political activism regarding child labor conditions.

    c. opposition to using untrained nursing aids to assist with World War I casualties.

    d. position on the issue of birth control.

11. There were several landmark reports about medical and nursing education that brought about changes in nursing. Match the report with its focus listed in the right column.

    _____ Flexner Report   a. Resulted in the establishment of practical nursing

    _____ Goldmark Report   b. Brought accountability to medical education

    _____ Brown Report   c. Identified the need for greater professional competence in nursing, recommended moving nursing education from hospitals to the university setting

    _____ Institute of Research and Service in Nursing Education Report   d. Identified that hospital-based training programs placed the institution's needs above the students' needs

12. Which of the following nursing pioneers suggested the establishment of a national health insurance plan?

    a. Isabel Hampton Robb

    b. Lillian Wald

    c. Adelaide Nutting

    d. Mary Mahoney

13. The main reason for the growth of insurance plans in the 1920s was

    a. physician advocacy.

    b. the influence of Metropolitan Insurance Company.

    c. the Depression.

    d. pressure from hospitals.

14. In 1977, an amendment to Title XVIII of the Social Security Act resulted in

    a. veterans and their dependents receiving free medical care.

    b. nurse practitioners being paid directly for rural health clinic services.

    c. the establishment of nurse clinical specialists.

    d. the provision of federal funds to expand enrollments in schools of nursing.

15. The Joint Commission on the Accreditation of Healthcare Organizations (JCAHO) plays a direct role in the improvement of the quality of health care delivery in the United States by viewing quality as

    a. an outcome.

    b. procedure oriented.

    c. person centered.

    d. related to the ratio of uninsured to insured Americans.

16. The goals of increasing quality and years of life and eliminating health disparities is the focus of Healthy People 2010, a program conducted by

    a. the U.S. Public Health Service.

    b. the Centers for Disease Control.

    c. the Agency for Health Care Quality.

    d. the National Institutes of Health.

17. Factors that contribute to the current nursing shortage include

    a. an aging workforce and retirement among nurses.

    b. stagnating salaries and low job satisfaction.

    c. a myriad of professional options for women entering the workforce.

    d. All of the above are contributing factors.

Critical Thinking

18. Which personal quality that an early nursing leader possessed is most influential in directing your professional career path? How does this quality reflect your ideals and values?

CHAPTER 2

The Health Care Delivery System

1. A nurse is educating clients about potential health problems related to overeating. Education is an example of which level of health promotion activity?

   a. Secondary prevention

   b. Primary prevention

   c. Tertiary prevention

   d. Chronic care management

2. A physician who is reimbursed directly by an insurance company for services provided is being reimbursed by which of the following methods?

   a. Capitation

   b. Fee-for-service

   c. Single-payer reimbursement

   d. Global payment system

3. One fundamental difference between the U.S. health care system and the Canadian health care system is that

   a. Canadians believe health care is a right for all and that, therefore, care is accessible to all.

   b. the U.S. system is more cost-effective in the way it delivers care.

   c. there is no difference; both systems offer all services to all people.

   d. U.S. citizens experience better health outcomes than Canadians.

4. Match the managed care model in the left column with its appropriate characteristic from the right column.

__b__	HMO (Health Maintenance Organization)	a. Care must be delivered by the plan in order for clients to receive reimbursement.
__c__	PPO (Preferred Provider Organization)	b. Focus on care is on cost-effective treatment measures with quality outcomes.
__a__	EPO (Exclusive Provider Organization)	c. Members are limited to providers within the system.

Copyright © 2004 by Delmar, a division of Thomson Learning, Inc. All rights reserved. **Chapter 2 • 5**

5. An issue that influences the quality of nursing care as increased nursing tasks are assigned to unlicensed assistive personnel (UAP) is the

    a. length of time UAPs are trained.

    b. character of the person filling the UAP role.

    c. educational level of the nurse responsible for the care of the client.

    d. quality of data the nurse uses in clinical decision making.

6. Managed care systems were developed to control

    a. ___access___

    b. ___cost___

    c. ___quality___

    of care before and during the delivery of services.

7. On which of the following health services is the most money spent in the United States?

    a. Medications

    b. Nursing home care

    c. Hospital care

    d. Physicians' services

8. Which of the following groups spurred the movement toward cost containment of health care?

    a. Physicians

    b. Insurance companies

    c. The business sector

    d. The American Association of Retired Persons (AARP)

9. Health care costs in the United States have escalated because

    a. there has been an increase in the numbers of HMOs.

    b. advances in technology allow more people to survive disabling diseases.

    c. there are an increased number of primary care providers in the marketplace.

    d. more people have access to health care providers today.

10. Identify three factors that are contributing to the nursing shortage.

   a. _____

   b. _____

   c. _____

11. The State Children's Health Insurance program passed by Congress in 1997

   a. provided health insurance to include all children regardless of parental income.

   b. expanded health insurance coverage for uninsured, low-income children.

   c. forced private insurers to broaden their definitions of covered children's diseases.

   d. included a provision for uninsured parents to be covered along with the child.

12. Which group is considered to be at the greatest risk for not having health care coverage?

   a. Middle-aged adults

   b. Children

   c. Elderly

   d. Disabled

13. Which of the following factors places the quality of hospital care at risk when hospitals restructure?

   a. Replacing brand-name medications with generic drugs

   b. Replacing RNs with UAPs

   c. Shortening the length of stay (LOS) for certain medical diagnoses

   d. Blending the roles of hospital workers into a multiskilled worker

14. The member of the health care team who is responsible for working with clients to enhance skills for activities of daily living is the

   a. physical therapist.

   b. nursing assistant.

   c. occupational therapist.

   d. chaplain.

15. In 1991 the nursing community put forth *Nursing's Agenda for Health Care Reform.* A cornerstone of this proposal is that

    a. all citizens must have access to health care services.

    b. health care services should be paid for by a single payer from public funds.

    c. health care must emphasize illness cure.

    d. integrated health systems must improve the continuity of care.

16. Which of the following statements would be accurate about nurse practitioner versus physician care?

    a. Nurse practitioners charge more for service.

    b. Nurse practitioners spend more time with their clients.

    c. Nurse practitioners can independently diagnose and resolve 80% of primary health problems.

    d. Nurse practitioners have prescriptive privileges in all states.

17. Subacute care emphasizes

    a. high acuity care.

    b. home care.

    c. curative interventions.

    d. restorative interventions.

Critical Thinking

18. A 19-year-old pregnant client is unemployed. She expresses concern about being able to get health care services for herself and for her unborn child. Describe the nurse's role in assisting this client. Identify options that are available and discuss how the client will access the health care system.

CHAPTER 3

Framework of Nursing Practice

1. Match the definitions from the right column with the terms in the left column.

    _____ concept

    _____ phenomenon

    _____ proposition

    _____ theory

    _____ discipline

    _____ research

    a. The use of formalized methods to generate information about a phenomenon

    b. A relational statement that links concepts

    c. Basic building block of theory

    d. Field of study

    e. An observable fact that can be perceived through the senses and explained

    f. Describes, explains, or predicts situations

2. Nursing practice, theory, and research exist

    a. independently of each other.

    b. as a closely related whole.

    c. in a loosely linked relationship.

    d. on a time-space continuum.

3. Which of the following would represent a grand nursing theory?

    a. Peplau's Theory of Interpersonal Relations

    b. Orem's Self-Care Deficit Theory of Nursing

    c. Nightingale's Notes on Nursing

    d. Abdellah's 21 Nursing Problems

4. Nursing theory development and research activities are directed toward

    _____.

5. The unifying force in a discipline that names the phenomena of concern to that discipline is called a

   a. paradigm.

   b. metaparadigm.

   c. framework.

   d. model.

6. Middle-range theories in nursing are

   a. used to describe complex relationships among many variables and to explain client situations.

   b. abstract and therefore best used to explain multiple events in nursing education.

   c. concrete and narrowly defined phenomena of interest to nurses.

   d. those that are derived exclusively from systematic inquiry using the scientific method.

7. According to Fawcett, the major concepts that provide structure to the domain of nursing are

   a. client, environment, health, nursing.

   b. nursing, client, environment, health.

   c. person, environment, nursing, well-being.

   d. person, environment, health, nursing.

8. The theorist who defines the paradigm of person as "more than the sum of the parts and is constantly changing . . . co-creating health through mutual interchange with the environment" is

   a. Martha Rogers.

   b. Rosemarie Parse.

   c. Imogene King.

   d. Sr. Callista Roy.

9. Which of the following nursing theorists put forward the following definition of nursing? "The unique function of the nurse is to assist the individual, sick or well, in the performance of those activities contributing to health or its recovery (or to peaceful death) that he would perform unaided if he had the necessary strength, will, or knowledge."

   a. Florence Nightingale

   b. Jean Watson

   c. Myra Levine

   d. Virginia Henderson

10. Mr. O'Grady is recovering from an aortic aneurysm repair. His recovery is complicated by a residual difficulty in swallowing, possibly secondary to a minor CVA during surgery. The speech therapist has placed him on a swallowing protocol, whereby he is relearning how to swallow. As a nurse, you are supporting this adaptive behavior, which fosters optimal functioning. Which of the following theories would best describe the theoretical framework you will be operating through as you support his coping?

    a. Orem's Self-Care Deficit Theory of Nursing

    b. The Roy Adaptation Model

    c. Watson's Theory of Human Caring

    d. Newman's System Model

11. Which of the following nursing theorists is concerned with a humanistic-altruistic philosophical basis for the science of nursing as well as the classification of caring behaviors?

    a. Jean Watson

    b. Martha Rogers

    c. Rosemarie Parse

    d. Dorothea Orem

12. Nursing borrows and uses theories from other disciplines. An example of a non-nursing theory is Maslow's Hierarchy of Basic Human Needs.

    ❑ True

    ❑ False

13. In a conversation with two nurse colleagues, you hear a discussion about the scope of practice of the various helping disciplines. When discussing the difference between medicine and nursing, Nurse A says medicine and nursing share the same metaparadigm, citing that nurses carry out doctors' orders. Nurse B states that the metaparadigm of nursing is broader than that of medicine. Which of these nurses represents the perspective aligned with current nursing theory and practice?

    a. Nurse A

    b. Nurse B

14. The concept of homeostasis becomes obsolete when considering the theory of which of the following theorists?

    a. Jean Watson

    b. Dorothea Orem

    c. Martha Rogers

    d. Sr. Callista Roy

15. General explanations that scientists and scholars use to explain, control, predict, and understand relationships among multiple events and variables are known as

    a. conceptual frameworks.

    b. theories.

    c. conceptual models.

    d. decision pathways.

16. Gordon's Functional Health Patterns theory is

    a. a tool used to predict behavior in clients with acute illnesses.

    b. a systematic holistic approach to evaluating client-care needs.

    c. an example of a grand theory used in a community practice setting.

    d. an integrated medical and nursing model of care.

17. Existentialism influenced the work of this early nursing theorist who focused her work on the human-to-human relationship and the meaning in experiences such as illness. Who was this theorist?

    a. Joyce Travelbee

    b. Faye Abdellah

    c. Myra Levine

    d. Patricia Benner

18. Whose nursing theories are consistent with the Simultaneity Paradigm?

    a. Martha Rogers

    b. Myra Levine

    c. Dorothea Orem

    d. Sr. Callista Roy

19. Mr. Hill, 38 years old, is a newly diagnosed diabetic. Since he is to be discharged tomorrow, you are reviewing aspects of his self-care regimen. You teach, reinforce, and ask for a demonstration of his ability to self-administer insulin injections. At the completion of the teaching session, he asks you to return later to review how to draw up insulin in a syringe. Which of the following theories would best describe the theoretical framework you will be operating through as you meet his self-care need?

    a. Orem's theory

    b. Watson's theory

    c. Levigne's theory

    d. Benner's theory

Critical Thinking

20. As a recent graduate you are excited about applying the theories you have learned in the practice setting. When you question a colleague about which theory the institution uses, she replies, "We don't use any nursing theory. It really is not that helpful in the real world." How would you respond to this nurse?

CHAPTER 4

The Nurse-Client Relationship

1. The purpose of using therapeutic communication is to

   a. create a beneficial outcome for the client.

   b. provide information to other professionals for diagnosing.

   c. obtain a health history.

   d. establish an intimate relationship with the client.

2. Match the component of the communication process in the left column with the definition of the term in the right column.

   _____ sender   a. Can be verbal or nonverbal

   _____ message   b. Generates messages

   _____ channel   c. Received as a reaction to a message

   _____ receiver   d. Intercepts messages

   _____ feedback   e. Can be auditory, visual, or kinesthetic

3. Match the type of personal space in the left column with a therapeutic example from the right column.

   __b__ intimate distance   a. Teaching a diabetes education class

   __c__ personal distance   b. Giving an injection

   __a__ social distance   c. Client demonstration of tube feeding

4. Which of the following best explains the importance of validating communication?

   a. Many clients with whom a nurse interacts are cognitively impaired.

   b. It assists a client with clarifying thoughts.

   c. Eye contact does not send the same message from culture to culture.

   d. Perceptions influence the interpretation of a message.

5. Which is an example of a closed-ended question?

    a. "Describe how the injury occurred."

    b. "How did you come to choose this clinic?"

    c. "Can you tell me where the pain is located?"

    d. "How have you been feeling lately?"

6. Which of the following is a characteristic of effective feedback? It is

    a. general vs. specific.

    b. independent of time.

    c. best delivered in a small-group setting.

    d. clear and unambiguous.

7. The nurse caring for an elderly client uses clear, easy-to-understand terms when explaining a procedure. This suggests the nurse understands that

    a. the client is elderly and probably won't understand medical terminology.

    b. simple, clear language is key to successful communication.

    c. the client must be experiencing Broca's aphasia.

    d. the family members are not well educated.

8. Match the type of group in the left column with the example from the right column.

    _____ self-help group   a. Commission on the nursing shortage

    _____ task group   b. Post-stroke management group

    _____ therapy group   c. Narcotics anonymous group

    _____ therapeutic group   d. Eating disorders group

9. Using a mannequin, the nurse discusses colostomy care and shows the client how to change a colostomy bag. The nurse hands the equipment to the client and asks for a return demonstration. Which communication channel(s) is the nurse using?

    _____

10. While transcribing medical orders to the medication administration record, the nurse notices that the route for a pain medication has been omitted. The nurse pages the physician and asks how the drug is to be given. The physician replies, "Give morphine sulfate 3mg intramuscularly, every 4 hours, as needed for pain." Which level of communication is being used in this situation?

    _____

11. The nurse is conducting the initial admission assessment on an 80-year-old client who is hearing impaired. Which communication skill should the nurse use to effectively communicate?

   a. Direct words to the client's hearing aid, while shouting.

   b. Speak slowly and face the client.

   c. Use a high-pitched voice while standing next to the client, who is seated in a chair.

   d. Perform only the physical assessment at this time.

12. The nurse is conducting a health history with a newly admitted client. Which nonverbal message sent by the nurse indicates openness, interest, and acceptance?

   a. Repeatedly tapping a pen on a clipboard while waiting for the client to reply.

   b. Sitting with arms folded and legs crossed while conducting the interview.

   c. Maintaining eye contact and leaning forward slightly while communicating with the client.

   d. Remaining expressionless when the client describes the recent loss of his spouse.

13. While initiating morning rounds, the nurse enters the room of a client scheduled for surgery and observes the client crying. Which behavior of the nurse reflects therapeutic communication?

   a. Patting the client's hand and telling the client not to cry.

   b. Telling the client that she'll return after she has finished morning rounds and checked her e-mail.

   c. Sharing a personal account of her own surgery and listing the similarities.

   d. Pulling a chair close to the client's bed and while sitting down stating, "I see that you are crying. Would you tell me why you are upset?"

14. Match the principles of therapeutic interactions in the left column with its outcome in the right column.

   _____ empathy   a. Sets the foundation of the therapeutic relationship

   _____ validation   b. Promotes understanding of the client's feelings and condition

   _____ active listening   c. Promotes truthfulness and sincerity

   _____ honesty   d. Promotes problem solving by the client

   _____ trust   e. Clarifies communication

15. A client tells the nurse that her son has been arrested again for drug possession and that this stress raises her blood pressure. The nurse's best response would be which of the following?

    a. "Have you tried joining Teen Challenge, a program for drug-addicted youth?"

    b. "A long stay in jail may be exactly what he needs."

    c. "Why don't you call a social worker—that discipline handles these problems."

    d. "What have you done before to cope with your son's problem?"

16. A nurse says, "Tell me about what concerns you most today." This request is an example of which of the following communication techniques?

    a. Broad opening statement

    b. Reflection

    c. Focusing

    d. Restating

17. Match the communication roadblock in the left column with its definition in the right column.

__c__	advising	a.	Pressuring the client to discuss something before he or she is ready
__d__	rejecting	b.	Statements that the nurse's views are those of the client
__b__	probing	c.	Offering the client direction about solving a problem
__e__	blaming	d.	Indicating to the client that certain topics are not open to discussion
__a__	agreeing	e.	Accusing the client of misconduct

18. Mrs. Alfonse, an 80-year-old widow, was admitted to your subacute facility two days ago from the local hospital, status post left-sided CVA. She cannot ambulate and has to be lifted to a chair. She has a pressure ulcer on her sacrum. As you redress it she states, "I can't believe I'm in a nursing home. What's going to become of me? I can't walk, I can barely feed myself, and I already have a sore on my bottom." Which of the following statements reflects a therapeutic response?

    a. "I'll leave a message for your doctor, so when she comes in she can talk about your progress."

    b. "That sounds like you are depressed. We can talk about it later."

    c. "You sound uncertain about your future. Tell me about your children who visited you yesterday."

    d. "Let me finish with this dressing and I'll get you fixed up and you'll feel better."

Critical Thinking

19. An elderly client who is no longer able to care for herself safely at home is being discharged to an assisted living facility. She is crying and states, "I just did not think I would ever have to give up my home." What can the nurse do to help the client?

20. What is self-talk? What impact does it have on the nurse-client relationship? What can the nurse to do promote successful communication?

CHAPTER 5 Culture and Ethnicity

1. Match the term in the left column with its definition from the right column.

   _____ culture

   a. The dynamic and integrated structures of knowledge, beliefs, behaviors, ideas, values, habits, customs, languages, symbols, rituals, ceremonies, and practices unique to a particular group of people

   _____ ethnicity

   b. A group that constitutes less than the majority of the population

   _____ race

   c. A group of people who have experiences different from the larger culture or society that functionally unifies the group

   _____ stereotyping

   d. The group whose values prevail within a society

   _____ dominant culture

   e. A grouping of people based on biological similarities

   _____ minority group

   f. Labeling people based on cultural preconceptions

   _____ subculture

   g. A cultural group's perception of themselves

2. There are six organizing factors nurses must consider when delivering culturally competent care: space, orientation to time, social organization, environmental control, biological variations, and _____.

3. Which conditions identified by the CDC are more prevalent among the poor?

   a. Obesity and hypertension

   b. Anorexia nervosa and sickle cell anemia

   c. Alzheimer's disease and stress fractures

   d. Lung cancer and multiple sclerosis

4. In which of the following cultural groups is eye contact considered a sign of disrespect?

   a. European American

   b. Native American

   c. Hispanic American

   d. African American

5. How should nurses support their clients' religious practices?

_____ .

6. In which of the following cultures does the family assume greater importance than the individual?

   a. Gay

   b. Middle-class European American

   c. Hispanic

   d. Upper-class European American

7. When caring for a client who does not speak English, using a qualified interpreter instead of a family member is desirable because

   a. the interpreter represents a neutral party.

   b. client confidentiality is maintained.

   c. the interpreter will be nonjudgmental and unbiased in translating sensitive information.

   d. All of the above are compelling reasons to use a qualified interpreter.

8. Which of the following best explains the purpose of the U.S. government WIC program?

   a. It provides destitute AIDS cases with supplemental income.

   b. It provides the homeless with shelter.

   c. It provides pregnant and breastfeeding mothers with supplemental food and other health services.

   d. It provides homeless children with food, shelter, and clothing.

9. Match the cultural group in the left column with its traditional healer from the right column.

   _____ African American   a. Herbalist

   _____ Asian American   b. Shaman

   _____ European American   c. Curandero

   _____ Hispanic American   d. "Community Mother"

   _____ Native American   e. Physician

10. What pediatric assessment tool, originally based on Eurocentric standards, underwent major revisions to reflect an ethnically diverse pediatric population?

_____

11. Which of the following approaches is essential to the delivery of culturally sensitive care?

   a. Technical competence

   b. Detailed knowledge of the client's culture

   c. A nonjudgmental attitude

   d. Fluency in the client's native language

12. Given that the incidence of tuberculosis is increasing, the knowledge of how isoniazid is metabolized differently among people of various cultural groups is important for the nurse to know. Which cultural groups metabolize isoniazid more quickly?

   a. European Americans, Asian Americans

   b. African Americans, Hispanics

   c. Native Americans, Asian Americans

   d. Hispanics, European Americans

13. Leininger's transcultural nursing theory is based on

   a. the concept that health and illness are determined by supernatural forces.

   b. the belief that illness results when one is not in harmony with the environment.

   c. the use of folk remedies and herbs to promote wellness.

   d. understanding cultural diversity and providing culturally competent care.

14. Culturally sensitive teaching guidelines include

   a. determining whether English is the client's primary language.

   b. assessing the client's level of education.

   c. including informed caregivers in the teaching process.

   d. asking the client and family what they need or want to learn.

   e. All of the above should be considered in the teaching process.

Critical Thinking

15. In some cultures babies do not sleep in a crib because their parents fear "crib death." Using Kleinman's Patient's Explanatory Model, develop a strategy the nurse would use with a caregiver who associates infant crib use with sudden infant death syndrome (SIDS).

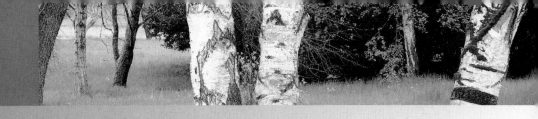

CHAPTER 6

Evidence-Based Practice and Nursing Research

1. The fundamental goal of research in nursing is to

    a. develop a body of knowledge that addresses medical problems.

    b. identify research priorities that will address and ameliorate the shortage of nurses.

    c. establish a credible body of evidence to support nursing care and improve practice.

    d. document the nurse's role as a primary care provider in the health care delivery system.

2. Which organization is considered to be responsible for coordinating and supporting research within the profession of nursing?

    a. American Nurses Association

    b. National Institute for Nursing Research

    c. National League for Nursing

    d. National Center for Nursing Research

3. Early research studies conducted by nurses focused on

    a. client satisfaction issues.

    b. disease prevention.

    c. nursing education.

    d. incident reports.

4. Which elements are considered essential components of an evidence-based practice model in nursing?

    a. Best research evidence, clinical expertise, and client values

    b. Clinical nursing expertise, client opinions, and medical research

    c. Integration of medical and nursing practice to provide good client care

    d. Clinical research, client evaluation of nurses, and nursing practice

5. Which action(s) would most likely lead to the implementation of evidence-based nursing practice?

   a. Efforts to change the behavior of the individual nurse

   b. The design of organizational systems that facilitate change

   c. Acceptance of nursing research by physicians

   d. Imposing standardized plans of care for all clients

6. Match the level of evidence from the left column with the type of research needed to support it from the right column.

   _____ Level 1

   _____ Level 2

   _____ Level 3A

   _____ Level 4

   a. Evidence obtained from at least one properly designed RCT

   b. Opinion of respected person, based on clinical experience, descriptive studies, or reports from expert committees

   c. Evidence obtained from a systematic review of relevant randomized control trials (RCT)

   d. Evidence from well-designed studies without randomization

7. A nursing research study that reports clinical observations and nursing activities during a 24-hour period would be considered

   a. descriptive.

   b. quantitative.

   c. ethnological.

   d. exploratory.

8. Which nursing research design uses methods that can be easily replicated and verified by others?

   a. Qualitative designs

   b. Quantitative designs

   c. Exploratory designs

   d. Hermeneutical designs

9. Which statement about the relationship of nursing practice to nursing research is most accurate?

    a. Research questions often arise from practice situations.

    b. Research does not have an impact on practice.

    c. There is a substantial body of nursing research that supports nursing practice.

    d. Researchers and clinicians disagree about how research should be conducted.

10. An example of nursing research that has made a significant contribution to nursing practice is to make nurses aware that

    a. teaching clients to perform daily finger sticks helps keep blood glucose levels under control.

    b. teaching clients the use of Kegel exercises, which strengthen pelvic floor muscles, decreases urinary incontinence in women.

    c. assisting physicians in the administration of multiple medications decreases the incidence of HIV infections.

    d. children who sleep with their parents are less likely to experience bad dreams than those who sleep alone.

11. The purpose of phenomenological research is to study

    a. causal relationships among multiple variables.

    b. social data in an effort to explain societal behaviors.

    c. individual, artifacts, and documents in their natural environments.

    d. the nature of human experience.

12. Which of the following type of research involves the systematic collection of numerical data, often under considerable control?

    a. Quantitative

    b. Qualitative

    c. Historical

    d. Ethnographic

13. Match the term in the left column with its definition from the right column.

    _____ hypothesis   a. Variation of a variable

    _____ independent variable   b. Statement of relationship between two variables

    _____ dependent variable   c. Abstraction inferred from situations or behaviors

    _____ construct   d. Outcome variable of interest

    _____ value   e. Controlled variable

14. When obtaining an informed consent from a client who is participating in a research study, the client is entitled to a full disclosure before signing a consent. This means that the client is informed about the nature of the study, the risks, and the benefits, as well as the right to refuse to participate.

❑ True

❑ False

15. Which of the following statements most accurately describes the role of the nurse without a graduate degree in the research process?

a. Designs research projects

b. Integrates research findings into care protocol changes

c. Collects research data as part of a research team

d. Acts as the principal investigator on a project

16. A research abstract is found at the beginning of a research article summarizing the purpose, methodology, findings, and conclusions of the study.

❑ True

❑ False

17. Increasing confidentiality of subjects can best be accomplished by

a. encrypting client data in computer programs.

b. avoiding collection of any personal identifying data.

c. refusing to let other researchers participate in the study.

d. All of the above

18. You are searching the Web for information on clinical practice guidelines that are designed to improve the quality of care on your unit. Which of the following Web sites would be most appropriate to consult?

a. *www.jacho.org*

b. *www.nlnac.org*

c. *www.aacn.nche.edu*

d. *www.joannabriggs.edu.au*

19. An article written by a nurse researcher is considered a(n)

    a. primary source.

    b. secondary source.

    c. tertiary source.

    d. original source.

Critical Thinking

20. On the nursing unit you are assisting with a research study assessing client reactions to the use of a new dressing material. A medical student questions the validity of nurses doing research. How would you respond?

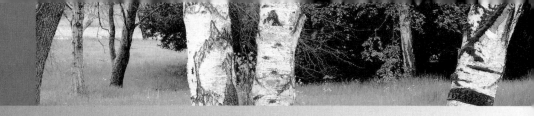

CHAPTER 7

Advanced Technology and Information Systems

1. Distance learning is best described as

   a. educational courses that integrate the Internet and computers in learning.

   b. educational courses offered only at satellite locations throughout a state or province.

   c. a curriculum of study that requires students to attend classes at a higher education campus on alternate weekends.

2. Give four examples of technologically sophisticated equipment that health care professionals use in the delivery of client care.

   a. _____

   b. _____

   c. _____

   d. _____

3. The handheld wireless computer device that is used in recording client information and for accessing reference material is called a

   a. pager.

   b. personal digital assistant.

   c. desktop computer.

   d. router.

4. Advantages of electronic health record documentation include

   a. the handwritten format, which contributes to legibility.

   b. that the client's record is accessible to all health team members without requiring a password.

   c. that the pharmacist can order medications and participate in medical treatment.

   d. that access to the record can be made from any point of service within the institutional system.

5. While a nurse is using a computerized medication administration record, a flag appears that advises the nurse to check the client's potassium level prior to giving the client a diuretic. The system that is assisting the nurse is called

    a. an expert system.

    b. a tracking system.

    c. a search engine.

    d. a spread sheet.

6. A protective mechanism that establishes limited access into a computer system is a

    _____.

7. The method of transmitting data or text files from one computer to another over an intranet or the Internet is

    a. spamming.

    b. electronic mail.

    c. text messaging.

    d. digital imaging.

8. Cite three ways in which portable computers assist community-based health care providers with client documentation.

    a. _____

    b. _____

    c. _____

9. Cite two cardiovascular monitoring devices that use computer technology.

    a. _____

    b. _____

10. List three chronic disease conditions in which telemonitoring services are directed.

    a. _____

    b. _____

    c. _____

11. Explain what a "virtual office visit" is.

    _____.

12. Soon many individuals will be carrying devices that store their insurance, medical, and health care information. This computerized apparatus is called a

    a. one card.

    b. ATM card.

    c. smart card.

    d. genome card.

13. The specialty in which nurses become expert in health care information technology is referred to as

    a. computer systems expert.

    b. advanced practice nursing.

    c. information specialist.

    d. nursing informatics.

14. Match the term in the left column with its descriptor from the right column.

    _____ cyberspace

    _____ listservers

    _____ networking computers

    _____ information superhighway

    _____ uniform resource locator

    a. Internet addresses used to locate information stored in specific computer bases

    b. The vast domain of all global Internet connections

    c. The infrastructure of the Internet that has been made possible through fiberoptic technology

    d. E-mail lists containing updated information on specific topics

    e. Computers connected to a central data storage base

Critical Thinking

15. Discuss the ways in which bedside computer systems used by health care providers can improve the delivery of health care.

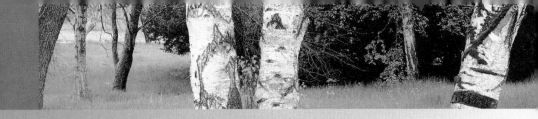

CHAPTER 8

Legal Accountability and Responsibilities

1. Which of the following mandates is the result of state administrative law action?

    a. Controlled Substances Act

    b. Nurse Practice Act

    c. Social Security Act

    d. National Labor Relations Act

2. Match the term in the left column with its definition in the right column.

    __c__ malpractice   a. Person being sued

    __b__ negligence   b. Breach of duty

    __d__ plaintiff   c. Wrongful conduct by a professional

    __a__ defendant   d. Party seeking damages

    __e__ testimony   e. Written or verbal evidence given by an expert in an area

3. Place the following elements for the proof of liability in the proper sequence.

    __3__ Injury is established.

    __4__ There was an obligation created by law, contract, or any voluntary action.

    __2__ A cause and effect is established linking the breach of duty to the injury.

    __1__ An act of omission or commission caused a breach of duty.

4. Under which of the following conditions is it legal to apply restraints?

    a. When a client is confused

    b. When a client is in danger of harming himself or harming others

    c. When a client is agitated

    d. When a client is threatening to leave the hospital against medical advice (AMA)

5. Which of the following actions by a nurse demonstrates an understanding of a client's right to privacy? The nurse

    a. checks on the client using the intercom.

    b. ensures the noise level in a client's room is kept to a minimum.

    c. knocks before entering a room.

    d. limits the visitors of a seriously ill client.

6. A nurse is overheard in the elevator discussing a neighbor, saying he was recently diagnosed with AIDS. This nurse can be held liable for

    a. slander.

    b. libel.

    c. fraud.

7. Issues of concern under the tenets of civil law include

    a. negligence and malpractice cases.

    b. refusal to enforce the use of the nursing process in delivery of care.

    c. basic civil rights of individuals and families.

    d. activities that interfere with normal functioning of a civilized society.

8. To what standard would a nurse be held when responding to an emergency in the community?

    a. By how a reasonable and prudent caregiver would have acted in the same situation.

    b. The nurse has full immunity from litigation.

    c. By the standards set forth in the local community hospital for emergency care.

    d. The nurse has full immunity as long as no money is accepted for the care rendered during the emergency.

9. A nurse is being charged with assault. This suggests the nurse committed which behavior?

    a. Touched the client, without consent, in a way that was harmful

    b. Threatened to administer an injection to keep the client quiet

    c. Failed to follow an incorrect medical order

    d. Allowed the nursing assistant to assess the client

10. You notice that a coworker's client has received three doses of narcotic analgesics throughout your shift, as documented on the MAR; however, the client continues to complain of pain. You remember that two days ago a similar occurrence happened when you worked with this colleague. You suspect that this person is signing out narcotic analgesics, documenting the analgesics were given, but not administering the analgesics to the patient. What should you do?

    a. Nothing

    b. Monitor the situation

    c. Report this coworker to the nursing supervisor

    d. Report this coworker to the State Board of Nursing

11. Which nursing action(s) would require the nurse to file an incident report?

    a. Administering the wrong medication to a client

    b. Placing a confused and combative client in restraints

    c. Referring the client's spouse to a social worker without the client's consent

    d. Counseling a client when family members are present

12. List four areas in nursing practice where nurses are at legal risk.

    a. _____

    b. _____

    c. _____

    d. _____

13. The physician has finished explaining a procedure and possible complications to the client and has allowed the client to ask questions about the procedure. The nurse is asked to witness consent to the procedure. By signing as a witness the nurse is assuring

    a. agreement with the necessity of the procedure.

    b. that the client understands the procedure and possible complications.

    c. that the client's signature is not a forgery.

    d. that the physician is the one performing the procedure.

14. A client falls and injures herself while under your care. Which of the following actions would you take to decrease the risk of liability to you?

    a. Document the incident carefully on an incident report form.

    b. Chart the facts surrounding the client's fall, client condition, and follow-up care.

    c. Do not document anything about the fall.

    d. Remove yourself as a caregiver for this client.

15. The Nurse Licensure Compact legislation was created to

    a. increase autonomy of baccalaureate-prepared nurses.

    b. allow for interstate nursing practice to occur.

    c. discourage nurses from traveling between geographical jurisdictions.

    d. remove disciplinary authority from the state in which the nurse is licensed.

16. In which of the following documents would a nurse seek to learn the name of the responsible person appointed by the client to make health care decisions when the client is unable to make his or her own health care decisions.

    a. Durable power of attorney

    b. Living will

    c. Advance care medical directive

    d. General consent form

17. Risk management programs are aimed at decreasing the risk of financial loss to the

    a. physician.

    b. agency.

    c. physician and nurse.

    d. agency, physician, and nurse.

18. Which of the following is the purpose of DNR physician's orders?

    a. To document the terminal nature of the client's condition

    b. To allow an alternative to the universal standing order to provide cardiopulmonary resuscitation to all clients

    c. To provide an opportunity for the patient, family, and caregivers to discuss the nature of the client's condition and the best possible course of action if the client has a cardiac arrest

    d. To provide legal protection for nurses who believe a client should not be resuscitated

Critical Thinking

19. A new graduate nurse working on your unit has not had time to purchase professional liability insurance. She asks you if it is really necessary to do so. How do you respond?

20. An elderly client is admitted to the unit from the emergency room. The nurse asks the nursing assistant to put the client in bed. The client gets in bed. The nursing assistant puts the siderails up and leaves the room. The client climbs over the siderails, falls, and sustains multiple fractures. Is the nurse liable for the client's injuries? Why?

1. Match the term in the left column with its definition from the right column.

   _e_ ethics
   a. The personal beliefs held by an individual that reflect religion or tradition

   _a_ morals
   b. What a person considers of worth, indirectly impacting behavior

   _b_ values
   c. The application of ethical principles to health care

   _d_ ethical principles
   d. Codes that direct or govern our actions

   _c_ bioethics
   e. The branch of philosophy that concerns the distinction of right and wrong on the basis of a body of knowledge

2. The statement, "The value of a situation is determined by its consequences" reflects which ethical theory?

   a. Deontology

   b. Bioethics

   c. Teleology

   d. Philosophy

3. The Nightingale Pledge states that while clients are under the care of a nurse, the nurse is to do no harm to the client. Which of the following ethical principles does this represent?

   a. Justice

   b. Nonmaleficence

   c. Fidelity

   d. Beneficence

4. Match the ethical principle in the left column with an appropriate example from the right column.

_b_   autonomy

_d_   nonmaleficence

_e_   beneficence

_f_   justice

_c_   veracity

_a_   fidelity

a. The nurse represents the client's viewpoint accurately during the interdisciplinary conference.

b. A client is asked to sign an informed consent form by a physician.

c. The nurse signs for a wasted narcotic only after she sees it being discarded.

d. The nurse triple checks the medication for "right medication and right dose."

e. The nurse considers whether a client should be physically restrained.

f. The client assignments on the unit are equally divided among the nurses.

5. Choosing not to work in a department where late-term terminations of pregnancies occur is a reflection of one's _moral values, religions belief_

6. List three frequently occurring ethical dilemmas in health care.

a. _Informed consent._

b. _Refusal of Tx_

c. _Incompetent health care provider._

7. Practicing nursing while under the influence of alcohol violates the American Nurses Association Code for Nurses. Which body has the authority to reprimand the nurse?

a. American Nurses Association (ANA)

b. Board of Nursing

c. National League of Nursing (NLN)

d. Commission on Collegiate Nursing (CCNE)

8. Which of the following is *not* included in the American Hospital Association (1992) "Patient's Bill of Rights"? The right to

a. considerate and respectful care.

b. make decisions about the plan of care.

c. have an advance directive concerning treatment.

d. sign a release of responsibility and leave the hospital at any time.

9. In which ways does the nurse act as a client advocate?

    a. By actively listening to a client's concerns

    b. By acting as a liaison between the client and other health care providers

    c. By educating clients about their individual health

    d. By convincing a client to participate in an experimental clinical trial

10. You are making an initial home care visit with Mrs. Lanscomb's nurse. Mrs. Lanscomb has recently been discharged from the hospital with a diagnosis of congestive heart failure and diabetes. After the assessment and interview, the nurse sits down with Mrs. Lanscomb and develops a plan of care to assist her in managing her medications and activities of daily living. Which of the following client rights is the nurse preserving?

    a. The right to make decisions regarding her care

    b. Her right to be involved in the treatment process

    c. The right to be treated with dignity and respect

    d. All of the above

11. In which of the following steps in the ethical decision-making process would the ethical dilemma be stated?

    a. Determination of claims and identification of parties

    b. Problem identification

    c. Generation of alternatives

    d. Assessing the outcome of moral actions

12. Which of the following best defines an ethical dilemma?

    a. A conflict between two or more ethical principles

    b. A conflict between the interests of two or more parties in the care of an individual

    c. A choice between two equally satisfactory alternatives

    d. A choice between the desired action of the nurse and the client

13. Match the term in the left column with its definition from the right column.

    ___d___ euthanasia   a. Taking deliberate action that hastens a client's death

    ___a___ active euthanasia   b. The omission of an action that would prolong a client's life

    ___b___ passive euthanasia   c. A health care professional providing the client with the means to end his or her own life

    ___c___ assisted suicide   d. The deliberate ending of a life as a human action

14. What is the ANA position on the participation of nurses in active euthanasia?

    a. Participation is in violation of nursing's ethical code.

    b. Participation is sanctioned only when the circumstances clearly warrant such action.

    c. Nursing's ethical code stands in support of active euthanasia.

15. Which of the following behaviors is unethical and illegal?

    a. Taking narcotics from the narcotic cabinet for your own use

    b. Assisting a physician in an abortion clinic to perform an abortion

    c. Allowing a gay (homosexual) AIDS client to sleep with his partner in the hospital

    d. Giving out client information over the telephone to a spouse

Critical Thinking

16. During an insertion of an introcath for IV therapy, an experienced nurse inadvertently punctures his finger with a sharp. The nurse immediately removes his gloves, washes the punctured site, and tells the client, whose HIV status is unknown, that he will draw a blood sample to be analyzed for any viruses. The client complies with the nurse's request but is reluctant to participate in further treatment. Are the nurse's concerns justified?

    Is it reasonable for a health professional to collect a blood sample from a client without the client's knowledge or consent?

    Is the nurse violating any ethical principle? Is the nurse violating the Patient's Bill of Rights?

    Could this situation be handled in a different manner?

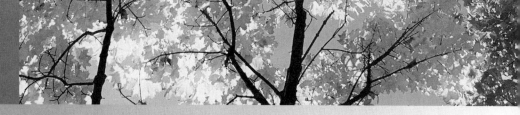

CHAPTER **10** **Critical Thinking and the Nursing Process**

1. Critical thinking can best be described as a process that

    _a._ is based on the problem-solving method.

    b. aims to make judgments based on evidence rather than on conjecture.

    c. uses intuition and knowledge gained from clinical situations.

    d. encompasses all of the above statements.

2. Match the characteristic of critical thinking on the left with its explanation on the right.

    ___c___ creativity   a. Anticipates an event, examines strategies to use

    ___a___ proactive   b. Uses reflective thought to analyze decisions

    ___d___ action-oriented   c. Explores new ideas and alternate ways to reach a conclusion

    ___b___ self-regulating judgment   d. Directed toward goal/resolution of a problem

3. Barriers to creative thinking include

    a. imagining and exploring alternatives.

    _b._ making decisions quickly without sufficient data.

    c. willingness to reconsider and explore change.

    d. being open-minded in evaluation.

4. Novice nurses develop clinical judgment as their length of time in nursing practice increases. Based on your understanding of critical thinking, which of the following statements is true about the development of clinical judgment?

    a. Clinical judgment develops at the same pace for every new nurse.

    b. New knowledge is unnecessary for clinical judgment to evolve.

    c. Exploration of alternative solutions to patient problems is not expected.

    d. An attitude of intellectual humility is the basis for questioning assumptions.

Chapter 10 • 45

5. A 5-year-old is brought to the ER by his mother. The child is audibly wheezing and using his accessory muscles to breathe. His respiratory rate is 38 breaths per minute. His mother tells the nurse that his asthma inhaler ran dry and that she hasn't had time to refill his prescription. Which need area takes priority in caring for this child?

    a. Noncompliance with drug therapy

    b. Knowledge deficit of asthma management

    c. Ineffective breathing pattern

    d. Risk for impaired parenting

6. Match the type of nursing diagnosis from the left column with its definition from the right column.

    _____ actual diagnosis   a. A potential client problem

    _____ risk diagnosis   b. A situation where a problem could exist if no action is taken

    _____ possible diagnosis   c. An existing client problem

    _____ wellness diagnosis   d. Reflects a situation in which a nurse manages the client's health status with a physician

    _____ collaborative diagnosis   e. Reflects a desire of the client to achieve a higher level of functioning

7. Write in the type of assessment data, either subjective data or objective data, on the lines provided.

    _____ S _____   "I'm short of breath."

    _____ O _____   Wound circular, 1½ inches in diameter, redness around edges, no drainage present

    _____ S _____   "I hear voices telling me to hurt myself."

    _____ O _____   Lung sounds clear bilaterally

    _____ S _____   "I am feeling upset now. I can't concentrate."

    _____ O _____   Vomited 150mL green-tinged fluid

8. The nursing diagnosis, "Alteration in skin integrity related to immobility as manifested by stage 1 pressure ulcer on coccyx," is an example of which of the following nursing diagnoses?

    a. Risk diagnosis

    b. Possible diagnosis

    c. Wellness diagnosis

    d. Actual diagnosis

9. As nurse Kelley reviews the client record for her assigned client, she reads the physician's orders for a client admitted to her unit with a diagnosis of pneumonia. Following this entry she reads down the list of treatments the physician has ordered. After she has assessed her client, she begins to write the nursing care plan for this client. She writes, "Ineffective airway clearance related to fatigue and weakness as manifested by inability to effectively cough and mobilize secretions." Reflect on the differences between the medical diagnosis and the nursing diagnosis. Which of the following statements is an accurate summary of the difference between a medical and a nursing diagnosis?

   a. The nursing diagnosis is determined by the medical diagnosis.

   b. The medical diagnosis is treated by the nurse.

   c. The nursing diagnosis reflects a human response to an actual problem.

   d. Only physicians can treat a pathophysiology.

10. The nurse asks the question, "Are there any risk factors here that could affect the health of my client?" Which phase of the nursing process is the nurse using?

   a. Assessment

   b. Diagnosis

   c. Implementation

   d. Evaluation

11. The nurse documents the following outcome goal on the care plan: "Client will ambulate 20 feet with walker, twice a day." The nurse has performed an activity in which of the following phases of the nursing process?

   a. Assessment

   b. Planning

   c. Implementing

   d. Evaluation

12. Expected outcome statements must be realistic, have a time limit, and be

   a. clear.

   b. broad.

   c. measurable.

13. When evaluating an elderly client's blood pressure reading, the nurse considers the client's age. In doing this, the nurse

    a. uses intuitive reasoning.

    b. compares data to geriatric norms.

    c. identifies gaps and inconsistencies.

    d. stereotypes the client by referring to developmental data.

14. The nurse develops the following outcome: "Stage II sacral pressure sore will improve within a week of prescribed therapy." What is wrong with this outcome?

    a. It does not have a time frame.

    b. It is not realistic.

    c. It is not appropriate.

    d. It is not measurable.

15. Thirty minutes after administering an oral analgesic, the nurse asks the client to rate his pain on a scale of one to ten. The nurse is engaging in which phase of the nursing process?

    a. Assessment

    b. Planning

    c. Implementing

    d. Evaluating

Critical Thinking

16. Each phase of the nursing process requires the nurse to use critical thinking skills. Beginning with assessment, examine relevant questions that reflect high-level thinking. Continue this exercise with each component of the nursing process.

1. Which best describes the difference between a focused and a comprehensive assessment?

   a. Comprehensive assessments are conducted as part of an initial examination, while focused examinations are conducted only after the client has been admitted to a unit.

   b. Focused examinations do not require any particular skill set on the part of a nurse, while comprehensive assessments require the expertise of an advanced clinician.

   c. Comprehensive assessments are illness related, while focused assessments are wellness oriented.

   d. Comprehensive assessments include collection of data about the whole person, while the focused assessments include data collection about a specific problem.

2. Your client arrives in the emergency room with a chief complaint of substernal chest pain. Which type of assessment is most appropriate when greeting the client?

   a. General

   b. Comprehensive

   c. Focal

   d. Ongoing

3. Which of the following aspects of a health history would a client most likely be reluctant to share with a nurse?

   a. Use of recreational drugs

   b. Use of herbal preparations

   c. Previous hospitalizations

   d. Prescription medications

Chapter 11 • **49**

4. The nurse's aide comes to you and states Mrs. Phillips says she has chest pain. Mrs. Phillips was admitted today with severe coronary artery disease and has a standard Heparin infusing at 860 units per hour. Her lab CPK results show no elevations and her EKG results show no new changes. What will be your first action when you see Mrs. Phillips?

   a. Ask her to describe the location, duration, and character of the pain.

   b. Administer the sublingual nitroglycerin ordered by the physician.

   c. Tell her that the pain is the result of the cardiac catheterization she experienced two days ago.

   d. Ask her to describe, in detail, her cardiac history.

5. Match the best assessment technique from the right column for determining the assessment finding in the left column.

   __B__ abdominal distention   a. Auscultation

   __A__ adventitious breath sounds b. Palpation

   __D__ circumoral pallor   c. Percussion

   __C__ lung tissue consolidation   d. Observation

6. During the interview the client states, "My right ear hurts off and on. Sometimes the pain is real sharp and I have to stop and wait for it to die down." Which of the following assessment techniques would the nurse use to gather objective data?

   a. Palpation

   b. Inspection

   c. Percussion

   d. Auscultation

7. The telemetry technician states Mr. Slayer's heart rhythm and rate has just changed from normal sinus rhythm with a heart rate of 78 to atrial fibrillation with a heart rate of 124. On his way to assess Mr. Slayer's vital signs the nurse obtains a sphygmomanometer. What important information will the nurse need prior to performing this assessment?

   a. The most recent EKG results

   b. The most recent CPK results

   c. A review of the client's past physical illnesses

   d. The baseline vital signs

8. The best source of data about the client is the

   a. family.

   b. client's records.

   c. physician.

   d. client.

9. Mrs. Jones presents with an oral temperature of 100 degrees F. Her chief complaint is frequency and burning upon urination. The nurse suspects that Mrs. Jones has a urinary tract infection. Which of the following assessments would validate the nurse's conclusion?

    a. Elevated WBC.

    b. Mrs. Jones is drinking large volumes of fluid.

    c. Elevated bacterial cell count of the urine.

    d. Mrs. Jones states, "When I have to go, I can't wait."

10. In what sequence would you expect to gather information about your hospitalized clients when you first begin your work shift?

    _6_ The medical record, the most recent lab work results

    _1_ The client

    _3_ The care plan, assessment flow sheets

    _2_ The nurses' shift report about the client

    _5_ The client's family

    _4_ Health care personnel

11. During the health interview the client reveals he gets stomachaches. The nurse asks him to describe what it feels like. The client states, "It feels like a train is racing through my gut." What type of information is the nurse seeking about the client's symptoms?

    a. Quality

    b. Aggravating factors

    c. Location

    d. Frequency

12. Mr. Kamal is due to be discharged within four days. He will need assistance with activities of daily living and will need to have a prothrombin time drawn twice a week. Which of the following questions would best elicit information needed to plan for his discharge needs?

    a. "What kind of assistance will you need in order to go to the laboratory to have your blood tests done?"

    b. "Will you need help at home?"

    c. "Will a family member help you at home?"

    d. "Do you have any assistive devices at home that will be of help to you?"

13. You have just heard a report on your client, Mrs. Smith, who has just returned from the OR after a cholecystectomy. She has an IV of D5 in 1/2 NS infusing at 100cc per hour, O_2 at 4L per nasal cannula, an NG tube attached to continuous low wall suction, and a Foley catheter. She has been medicated for incisional discomfort with 10mg of morphine sulfate sc one hour ago. The report revealed that Mrs. Smith is slightly nauseated. Her husband is in the room with her. Which of the following assessments is priority upon entering the room?

    a. The position of the siderails

    b. Assessment of the wound for drainage

    c. Check to see if the oxygen is set at the proper flow rate

    d. The temperature of the room

14. The expected outcome of the nursing assessment is

    a. the development of a comprehensive client database.

    b. an extensive systems review of all of the client's complaints.

    c. the development of a nursing diagnosis.

    d. a historical review of the client's prior illnesses.

15. Accurate documentation of client status is essential. Which documentation format would allow for consistency in recording data and flexibility of recording specific information?

    a. Checklists

    b. Open-ended

    c. Specialty

    d. Combination

16. Mr. Hays will be discharged on Digoxin 0.25mg po q A.M. You are planning to discuss this medication with him. After reviewing nursing considerations for this medication, select the interview question that would be most helpful in planning for his needs.

    a. "If your pulse is less than 50 beats per minute, what will you do?"

    b. "Where does this drug act on the body?"

    c. "Do you know what the side effects of Digoxin are?"

17. Mr. Daniels has just arrived on your unit to undergo surgery the next morning. You need to interview him in order to complete your nursing assessment. His roommate has several noisy visitors and the TV is on. Which of the following actions could you take in order to accomplish the interview?

    a. Close the curtain to provide privacy.

    b. Ask his roommate to turn down the volume of the TV.

    c. Escort Mr. Daniels to a private, quiet space if a suitable room is available.

    d. All of the listed actions

    e. None of the listed actions

Labeling Exercise

18. Which physical assessment technique is the nurse using? What kind of information will the nurse gain from using this technique?

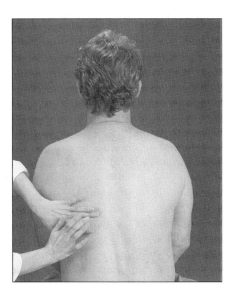

Critical Thinking

19. A 48-year-old client comes into the ER using an assistive device for ambulation. On initial inspection the nurse observes the client holding a bag of ice to the left foot. A friend informs the nurse that the client fell and is now unable to put weight on the affected foot and is experiencing pain. What type of assessment is warranted in this situation? What kind of information will the nurse want to obtain from the client?

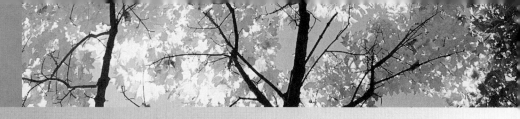

CHAPTER **12** **Nursing Diagnosis**

1. Nursing and medical diagnosis share some similar elements. Which statement reflects their commonality?

    a. Both focus on the pathological condition.

    b. Both use a logical systematic process to arrive at diagnoses.

    c. Both develop interventions and treatment based solely on the medical diagnosis.

    d. Both focus on the human response and the risk for developing conditions.

2. List the three contexts in which the nursing process is used.

    a. ___Data analysis___

    b. ___product/diagnosist label___

    c. ___organized classification___

3. Which of the following is best defined by the statement, "A clinical judgment about an individual, family, or community response to actual and potential health problems/life processes"?

    a. Nursing diagnosis

    b. Medical diagnosis

    c. Collaborative problem

    d. Independent problem

4. The first nursing diagnosis conference in 1973 began to identify, develop, and place nursing diagnoses in a taxonomy. Which of the following statements is correct about the nursing diagnosis taxonomy?

    a. It is a list of nursing diagnoses.

    b. It is a classification of human responses.

    c. It is a complete list of all possible diagnoses.

    d. Each nursing diagnosis has been validated using medical diagnoses as a standard.

5. Consider the following nursing diagnosis: *Ineffective Airway Clearance R/T fatigue as evidenced by dyspnea at rest*. Which portion represents the etiology for this diagnosis?

   a. Ineffective airway clearance

   b. Fatigue

   c. Dyspnea at rest

6. Which of the following statements are reasons why nurses should use NANDA-approved diagnoses?

   a. Nursing diagnoses may be linked to computerized documentation systems.

   b. Nursing diagnoses provide the basis for selection of nursing interventions.

   c. Nursing diagnoses guide outcome statements.

   d. Nursing diagnoses provide a common language for practice.

   e. All of these statements support the use of NANDA-approved diagnoses.

7. Which of the following type of nursing diagnosis identifies the individual or aggregate condition or state that may be enhanced by health-promoting activities?

   a. Actual

   b. Risk

   c. Wellness

   d. Syndrome

8. List in sequence the steps in developing a nursing diagnosis.

   __4__ Data is clustered.

   __6__ The first part of the diagnosis is written (diagnostic label).

   __3__ Data cues are interpreted and assigned meaning.

   __7__ Related to (R/T) factors are identified and attached to the diagnosis.

   __1__ Data cues are identified from client data.

   __2__ Data cues are validated.

   __5__ A list of nursing diagnoses is consulted.

9. Consider the nursing diagnosis *Acute Pain R/T pain from incision*. Which of the following statements identifies the error in this nursing diagnosis?

   a. It is saying the same thing twice.

   b. It is using a medical diagnosis in the nursing diagnosis.

   c. It is a judgmental statement.

   d. It should have been written as a one-part nursing diagnosis.

10. A client shares his desire to quit smoking. Which diagnosis reflects the client's desire to achieve this goal?

    a. Risk for lung cancer

    b. Readiness to engage in smoking cessation program

    c. Enhance well-being related to nicotine cessation

    d. Ineffective breathing pattern related to 30-pack-years of cigarette smoking

11. What is indicated when NANDA lists the word *specify* in parentheses, with certain diagnoses?

    It means include a descriptive qualifier
    It make your Dx clear.

12. Valuing is one of the nine human response patterns in which the taxonomy of nursing diagnoses is ordered. Which statement is related to *valuing*?

    a. To transmit thoughts or feelings

    b. To become aware through the senses

    c. To be emotionally affected by the experience

    d. To equate an importance

13. Match the human response pattern in the left column to the nursing diagnosis in the right column.

    _d_ choosing   a. Risk for constipation
    _c_ moving   b. Acute pain
    _e_ perceiving   c. Fatigue
    _b_ feeling   d. Disabled family coping
    _a_ exchanging   e. Hopelessness

14. List the components of the three-part nursing diagnosis statement.

    a. _Problem RT_

    b. _etiology_

    c. _defining characteristics_

15. The nurse develops the nursing diagnostic statement *Risk for aspiration related to difficulty with swallowing*. What is the risk factor?

    a. Dysphagia

    b. Malnutrition

    c. Aspiration

    d. Impaired dentition

16. Which strategy can the nurse use to avoid making common diagnostic errors?

    a. State the diagnosis to reflect medical conditions.

    b. Use only objective data in constructing the diagnostic statement.

    c. Recognize that an initial diagnosis is subject to change.

    d. Use a symptom reported by the client as the first part of the diagnostic statement.

17. Nursing outcomes classification (NOC) uses a scale to measure outcomes, which provide quantifiable information.

    ☑ True

    ❑ False

18. The nursing intervention classification (NIC) and the nursing outcomes classification (NOC) are recognized by

    a. JCAHO and the ANA.

    b. State Board of Nursing and NANDA.

    c. OMAHA and the National League of Nurses.

    d. CINAHL and Ovid databases.

Critical Thinking

19. Discuss three reasons why the nursing process is essential for nursing practice.

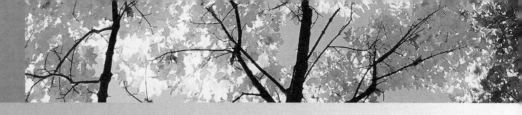

CHAPTER **13** **Outcome Identification and Planning**

1. Outcome identification and planning, essential components of the nursing process, are used as tools to

    a. alert physicians to changes in the client status.

    b. provide adequate direction to ensure the delivery of competent nursing care.

    c. direct nursing assistants and other health care providers to assist the nurse.

    d. provide information about the client's biopsychosocial history.

2. According to the ANA standards, which of the following is a criterion for the development of client expected outcomes?

    a. The outcome must be documented in measurable terms.

    b. The outcome must be comprehensive.

    c. The outcome must be setting specific.

    d. The outcome must be approved by an outside reviewer.

3. Match the term in the left column with its definition from the right column.

    _____ initial planning   a. An expectation to be achieved in a few days or hours

    _____ ongoing planning   b. The plan developed for the client's care upon leaving the facility

    _____ discharge planning   c. The continuous updating of the client's plan of care

    _____ short-term goal   d. The plan developed as a result of the admission assessment

    _____ long-term goal   e. An expectation to be achieved in weeks or months

4. Prioritize the following nursing diagnoses from *high* to *low*.

    _____ Hyperthermia

    _____ Risk for impaired skin integrity

    _____ Spiritual distress

5. Mr. Butterworth has been hospitalized for three days. When you enter his room to do the daily assessment, he asks you if he could be shaved today, citing that he has been unshaven since his admission. Which of the following is the best response?

   a. "I'm sorry, I do not have time today to shave you."

   b. "I will see if I can fit this into your plan of care for today. Let me get back to you."

   c. "I understand your need to be shaved; it will make you feel better. I will see to it that you get a shave."

   d. "Is your wife coming in today? Possibly she can shave you."

6. The nurse develops a diagnosis of ineffective tissue perfusion for a client with a medical diagnosis of peripheral vascular disease. Identify the most appropriate short-term expected outcome for a client with this diagnosis.

   a. The client will have palpable peripheral pulses in 2 weeks.

   b. The client will identify three ways to improve peripheral circulation.

   c. The client will experience increased sensation in his feet and toes.

   d. The client will optimize his circulation by walking 1 mile q day.

7. Which of the following terms does *not* describe a goal statement?

   a. It is measurable.

   b. It is written in current or past tense.

   c. It specifies a time frame for the task accomplishment.

   d. It is realistic for the client.

8. Which of the following type of nursing order is "Teach the client the importance of adherence to a low-fat diet"?

   a. Health promotion

   b. Prevention

   c. Observation

   d. Treatment

9. Which of the following would be an example of a client need where the nurse would call a consultation?

   a. The client is immobile and at risk for a break in skin integrity.

   b. The client has a knowledge deficit regarding ambulation with crutches on a flat surface as well as climbing stairs.

   c. The client has a Foley catheter and a primary IV infusing and is at risk for infection.

   d. The client is confused and frail with a history of falls and is at risk for injury.

10. In the following goal statement, which portion is the *task statement*? "The client will ambulate the entire length of the hallway three times by Friday."

    a. The client

    b. Will ambulate

    c. The entire length of the hallway

    d. By Friday

11. Which statement includes a set of conditions by which a client will accomplish expected outcomes?

    a. By Friday, the client will ambulate 30 feet three times with the use of a walker.

    b. The client will ambulate 30 feet three times a day.

    c. The client will demonstrate the technique for self-administration of heparin.

    d. By Wednesday, the client will perform a breast self-exam.

12. After developing the nursing diagnosis *Pain (chronic) related to bilateral inflammation of knee and hip joints*, the nurse develops a list of interventions directed at alleviating the client's pain. Which phase of the nursing process is the nurse focused on?

    a. Diagnosing

    b. Planning

    c. Implementing

    d. Evaluating

13. Which element of a nursing order is missing in the following statement? "9/27/2003: Auscultate apical pulse prior to administering Digoxin 0.25mg. *B. Griffin RN*"

    a. Date

    b. Action verb

    c. Detailed description

    d. Time frame

    e. Signature

14. What criteria is missing from the following short-term outcome statement? "The client will ambulate 20 feet with a walker."

    a. Time frame

    b. Measurable performance

    c. Client behavior

    d. Condition or qualifier

15. Mrs. Langly is a 45-year-old client who has a history of diabetes, end-stage renal disease, and peripheral vascular disease. She was admitted to your unit for unstable blood levels of BUN, creatinine, and glucose. Which of the following goals would be appropriate for Mrs. Langly?

    a. The client will plan a low-protein, 1,800-calorie diabetic diet for 48 hours by Friday.

    b. The client will demonstrate effective coping by discharge.

    c. The client will be able to plan for an appropriate diet by Thursday.

    d. The client will know why it is important to follow a diet by discharge.

16. Consider the following nursing diagnosis for a one-day post-op client: *Risk for Infection R/T surgical incision.* Which of the following interventions would be appropriate for this nursing diagnosis?

    a. Assess wound for signs of redness or drainage q shift.

    b. Assess IV site for inflammation or infiltration.

    c. Change steri strips q shift, assess wound.

    d. Monitor pulse rate q 4h.

17. Consider the following nursing diagnosis for a client who is on bedrest: *Risk for Altered Respiratory Function R/T stasis of secretions secondary to immobility.* Which of the following nursing interventions on the care plan was derived from the etiological portion of the nursing diagnostic statement?

    a. Offer the client a back rub q shift.

    b. Encourage client to do leg exercises q 2h.

    c. Assist client to turn, deep breathe, and cough q 2h.

    d. Suction oral secretions PRN.

Critical Thinking

18. A 56-year-old male, who was having acute chest pain, was brought to the ER by his wife. He was sweating heavily, was short of breath, and stated that he felt nauseous. While the triage nurse was taking his vital signs, his cell phone rang. He asked his wife to hand him the phone, as it was a call from an important customer. The nurse intervened and attended to his most immediate need.

    Using Maslow's Hierarchy of Basic Human Needs, prioritize the client's problems. Which problems require immediate intervention? Does the client have needs that can be attended to later?

1. At the beginning of a work shift a nurse establishes a shift worksheet considering client care priorities. Which of the following would be placed on the shift worksheet first?

   a. Medication administration

   b. Client assessments

   c. Care plan reviews

   d. Vital sign measurements

2. The transfer of tasks to an individual who is competent in performing these tasks is called

   a. delegation.

   b. management.

   c. validation.

   d. task segmentation.

3. Match the type of nursing management system in the left column with its definition in the right column.

   _____ functional nursing   a. The RN is the leader; LPNs care for acutely ill clients; nursing assistants serve trays and assist with ADLs.

   _____ team nursing   b. The RN assumes responsibility for client care and coordination of care regardless of the location of the client.

   _____ primary nursing   c. Caregivers are assigned to a segment of the client-care unit.

   _____ modular nursing   d. Care is divided into tasks and each person assumes a task.

   _____ case management   e. The RN assumes responsibility for total client care.

4. Which of the following care management systems is the most costly to maintain?

   a. Team nursing

   b. Modular care

   c. Case management

   d. Primary nursing

5. Which of the following statements is true about nursing interventions? They are

   a. actions that help clients achieve goals.

   b. written broadly, not specifically.

   c. exclusively dependent on physicians' orders.

   d. written as a goal statement.

6. An example of an independent nursing intervention is

   a. administering intravenous fluids for a client diagnosed with nutritional impairment.

   b. turning and repositioning a client with impaired mobility every 2 hours.

   c. ordering a chest x-ray for a client diagnosed with ineffective breathing pattern.

   d. reviewing laboratory values and reordering tests for abnormal values.

7. Which of the following is considered an example of a standing physician's order?

   a. A protocol for indwelling urinary catheter care

   b. Hemoglobin and hematocrit two days postpartum on all postpartum patients

   c. The procedure for the flush of peripherally inserted central line catheters

   d. A skin care protocol for a client who is immobile

8. Identifying and understanding rationales for nursing interventions are integral to the development of the client plan of care. Which of the following best describes a rationale?

   a. Theory

   b. Pathophysiological condition

   c. Fundamental principle

   d. Nursing measure

9. The standardized nursing language that offers the profession of nursing the potential for direct reimbursement of services is

   a. NIC.

   b. NOC.

   c. NANDA.

   d. ANA.

10. Outcome criteria are

    a. the same as goals.

    b. used to determine whether a goal has been met.

    c. determined by the client.

    d. used only when planning short-term care.

11. You are to administer an IV medication. Your client has total parenteral nutrition (TPN), lipids, and a minibag of potassium (KCl) supplement infusing through separate IV lines. After preparing the IV medication you enter the client's room and are unsure which IV line to use to administer the medication. What should you do?

    a. Call the pharmacy for help.

    b. Ask a fellow student nurse for an opinion.

    c. Seek the assistance of the staff nurse assigned to your client.

    d. Use the IV line that is infusing the TPN.

12. The class of nursing interventions Electrolyte and Acid-Base Balance falls into which of the following domains of the Nursing Intervention Classification?

    a. Physiological: Basic

    b. Physiological: Complex

    c. Safety

    d. Health System

13. Using aseptic techniques, a nurse demonstrates insulin preparation to a client. This is an example of which phase of the nursing process?

    a. Assessing

    b. Implementing

    c. Diagnosing

    d. Planning

14. Which of the following nursing interventions is considered a skilled therapeutic intervention?

    a. Assisting a client to ambulate with a walker

    b. Feeding a client who has difficulty swallowing

    c. Bathing a client who is confused

    d. Administering a medication to a client who is hypertensive

15. Which of the following is expected of a nurse after carrying out a nursing intervention?

    a. Notifying the physician of completion of the intervention

    b. Explaining to the client the reason for the intervention

    c. Reassessing the client

    d. Teaching the family the expected outcomes

16. Which of the following would create an opportunity for the nurse to teach a client?

    a. Medication administration

    b. Vital sign measurement

    c. Changing a wound dressing

    d. All of the above

17. When a task is delegated, the role of the nurse is to

    a. validate the skill level of the care provider.

    b. assume the task was completed as expected.

    c. allow the care provider independence during task completion.

    d. review care provider notes.

18. Developing psychomotor goals for the physically impaired client allows the nurse to

    a. determine how much knowledge the client has retained after being taught the side effects of a medication.

    b. measure the client's ability to perform certain activities.

    c. communicate the client's needs with family and other health care providers.

    d. assess client's feelings about limitations.

Critical Thinking

19. When reviewing a chart, the nurse notes that the PCA has been documenting client responses to nursing interventions for which the nurses are responsible. When questioned, the PCA states that the evening nurse needed help finishing the charts on time. How would you handle this situation? What is the nurse's responsibility for delegation and documentation?

1. Check all of the following behaviors that apply to the evaluation of nursing care.

    ____a. Establishing the initial database for a client as a result of the admission assessment

    ____b. Juxtaposing the client's response against an expected outcome

    ____c. Inviting the parents of a pediatric client to discuss the progress of their child toward an expected outcome

    ____d. Interpreting a cardiac rhythm strip

    ____e. Determining whether an objective on the care plan was achieved by the client

    ____f. Asking the client what he or she would like to achieve as an outcome of treatment

2. Which of the following outcomes would you expect as a result of a nursing audit?

    a. Revision of the facility mission and philosophy statement

    b. Revision to the standards of care related to the prevention of falls

    c. Revision to the care plan of an individual client

    d. Revision of the job description of the unlicensed assistive personnel (UAP)

3. In which of the following phases of the nursing process is the evaluation process reflected?

    a. Assessment and implementation

    b. Assessment and diagnosis

    c. Outcome identification and implementation

    d. Assessment, diagnosis, planning, and implementation

4. You review the RN staff nurse job description at Mercy Hospital for accuracy, keeping in mind that the establishment of job descriptions is one mechanism the hospital uses to deliver quality outcomes. Which of the following describes the type of evaluation you are conducting?

    a. Structural

    b. Process

    c. Outcome

5. Which of the following evaluation methods reflects a process evaluation?

    a. The assistant manager asks you to review the client records of the last 10 clients discharged for documentation of client response to analgesics administered.

    b. The division director asks you to make rounds on all the client care units to see if the nursing policies are easily accessible.

    c. The evening supervisor asks you to analyze the staffing patterns for the evening shift to determine whether staffing is adequate to meet the acuity needs of clients.

    d. The case manager for your client asks you to determine whether the client's discharge goal related to knowledge deficit has been met.

6. A _____ evaluation is used to measure the adequacies of nursing activities in implementing the nursing process.

7. Which of the following would you monitor as an indicator of quality care?

    a. The level of your clients' functionality at the time of discharge

    b. The satisfaction of the physicians on your unit with the nursing care delivered at your facility

    c. The results of the client satisfaction survey that pertain to your unit

    d. The level of client comorbidity at the time of admission to your unit

8. During rounds, Mrs. Jones's physician asks you if Mrs. Jones has met the expected outcome of ambulating around the unit four times a day with minimal assistance. What primary data source would you consult before you answer the physician?

    a. The client record

    b. The family

    c. The UAP

    d. The client

9. You determine that your client has not met an expected outcome. What action do you take?

    a. Call a meeting of the interdisciplinary team.

    b. Ask the client why the goal was not accomplished.

    c. Call for a nursing consultation.

    d. Review and revise the care plan.

10. Evaluation is based primarily on

    a. information retrieval and documentation.

    b. observation and communication.

    c. effective use of the nursing process.

    d. delivery of nursing care and analysis of client goals.

11. An aspect of evaluation that provides a basis for autonomy and self-governance for nursing practice is

    a. the application of agency standards.

    b. the peer evaluation process.

    c. multidisciplinary collaboration.

    d. the application of union rules to nursing practice.

12. Evaluation of a client's progress toward a stated outcome should occur

    a. at the time of intervention.

    b. on discharge from the institution.

    c. on completion of treatment.

    d. only when progress is evident.

13. The nurse develops a diagnosis of knowledge deficit related to self-care of an open wound. One outcome criteria identified is that after the first session with the nurse, the client will be able to gather the necessary equipment for self-care. The client gathers most of the equipment but forgets sterile gloves. Which of the following evaluative statements should the nurse write?

    a. Goal not met: Client unable to get all of the materials needed for a dressing change.

    b. Goal partially met: Client gathers most of the supplies needed.

    c. Goal not met: Client able to gather all supplies except sterile gloves.

    d. Goal met: Client gathered most of supplies and was able to tell nurse which ones were missing.

14. A nursing audit is used to evaluate

    a. the nursing process.

    b. institutional standards.

    c. quality of nursing care.

    d. client outcomes and goal achievement.

15. The purpose of evaluation in the nursing process is to

    a. determine whether a client's problems are resolved.

    b. determine whether the nurse developed independent outcome criteria for the client.

    c. select appropriate nursing goals and objectives.

    d. develop a time frame for completing the nurse-client relationship.

Critical Thinking

16. A 65-year-old client diagnosed with type 2 diabetes mellitus will be discharged home from the hospital within 2 days of admission. The nurse determines the client needs teaching related to diet, activity, and oral medication management. When should evaluation begin? What impact will evaluation have on the nursing interventions?

CHAPTER 16 Documentation and Reporting

1. Standards regulating client access to his or her medical records are controlled by

    a. state regulatory bodies.

    b. hospital and physician practice standards.

    c. federal legislation and subsequent regulation.

    d. the Patient's Bill of Rights.

2. Which of the following is the best defense of a nurse during a malpractice lawsuit?

    a. Depositions by fellow nurses

    b. The client record

    c. Character witnesses

    d. Personal anecdotal notes

3. Which of the following statements best describes the information contained in the consultation sheet found in the medical record?

    a. It contains medical orders and the treatment plan.

    b. It contains a record of the client's vital signs.

    c. It contains a record of the history and physical examination conducted by the attending physician.

    d. It contains a request for the services of other practitioners.

4. While reviewing a client record, you come upon a form that includes information about the client's wishes regarding life-sustaining procedures if the client becomes unable to make these decisions. This form is a(n)

    a. durable power of attorney for health care.

    b. advance directive.

    c. informed consent.

    d. incident form.

5. Which of the following statements best interprets the signature on an informed consent form by a nurse as witness to the client's signature?

   a. The client understands the procedure written on the consent form.

   b. The physician has explained the procedure to the client.

   c. The client is, in fact, the client and is competent to make a decision.

   d. The nurse was assigned to the client at the time of obtaining the informed consent.

6. How would the following narrative charting entry be considered? "3/28/03 9:15 A.M. Awake, tolerated little sips of water. Skin, warm and moist to touch. Mild anxiety noted. K, Camp, RN."

   a. Well written and accurate

   b. Unsatisfactory; data are nonspecific.

   c. Satisfactory; data are complete and relevant to client situation.

   d. Okay for a narrative entry.

7. Documentation of assessment, intervention, and evaluation of client status and response to treatments should be done

   a. at the end of the nursing shift.

   b. right before the treatment or medication is administered.

   c. at least two to three times each shift.

   d. as close as possible to the actual time the activities occur.

8. Which of the following statements depicts the correct action to take if you make a documentation mistake on the medical record?

   a. Erase the mistake and write over it.

   b. Scratch it out so it is completely obliterated.

   c. Cross it out and go on with the recording.

   d. Draw one line through it, and sign and date the correction.

9. Which of the following organizations approves abbreviations and symbols for use in a medical record?

   a. ANA

   b. AMA

   c. NANDA

   d. The health care organization

10. Match the method of documentation in the left column with its example or definition from the right column.

_____ narrative charting

_____ problem-oriented medical record

_____ PIE charting

_____ focus charting

_____ charting by exception

_____ computerized documentation

a. SOAP note entries are made in the medical record.

b. Saves documentation time, increases legibility, and facilitates the statistical analysis of data.

c. Flow sheets are used extensively; deviations from preestablished norms are documented.

d. Uses a chronological, storytelling format.

e. Charting uses a columnar format within the progress notes to distinguish it from other recordings in the narrative notes.

f. Incorporates the ongoing plan of care into the daily charting.

11. You accompany a home care nurse making a home visit. After leaving the home the nurse enters client data into a handheld computer. Which of the following best describes this documentation system? It is

a. point-of-care charting.

b. focus charting.

c. narrative charting.

d. None of the above

12. Which of the following nurse's note entries in the medical record is most accurate?

a. Pt. is able to deep breathe and cough without difficulty.

b. Pt. performs deep breathing and coughing exercises independently; cough is nonproductive.

c. Pt. assisted with deep breathing and coughing (DB&C) exercising, expectorating small amounts of clear sputum. Lung sounds clear after DB&C activity.

d. Pt. states deep breathing and coughing exercises are painful.

13. Which of the following is a necessary element in order for computerized documentation systems in health care agencies to demonstrate the quality, effectiveness, and value of nursing service?

a. A standardized nursing language

b. Standardized databases

c. A final version of the nursing taxonomy

d. Nurses who are able to improve client care delivery systems

14. Which of the following is the most accurate entry on the physician's order sheet by a nurse after taking a telephone order from a physician?

    a. Give Lasix 40mg IVP now
       T.O. Dr. Donohue/Mary Smith RN

    b. Verapamil 5mg IVP stat
       Dr. Jones/Mary Smith RN

    c. Dulcolax tablets for constipation
       Dr. Cordovan/Mary Smith RN

    d. Tylenol 650mg q 4–6h PRN for headache
       Mary Smith RN

15. It is recommended that nurses document a client incident of a fall carefully on the client record. Which of the following is the correct rationale for this?

    a. Falls are costly to treat.

    b. Falls are the main reason nurses are sued.

    c. The data is used by risk managers to identify factors that create risk for falls in a client population in a facility.

    d. The documentation assists the physician with diagnosing and treating the client's condition after the fall.

16. Which of the following documentation systems would the nurse be expected to use to document a variance from an expected outcome?

    a. Narrative charting

    b. Charting by exception

    c. Critical pathway

    d. Nursing care Kardex

Critical Thinking

17. As a new RN you are assigned to a preceptor on your unit. You observe the nurse charting treatments and medications prior to actual administration and implementation. Is this appropriate behavior? What are the implications of the behavior? How would you handle the situation?

1. Which of the following statements accurately reflects the principles of growth and development?

    a. Development occurs in a caudalcaphalo direction.

    b. Functions closer to the midline of the body develop before functions farther away from the body's midline.

    c. Development proceeds from complex to simple and general to the specific.

    d. Passage through developmental stages occurs within a specific time schedule.

2. The period of infancy is defined as

    a. 32 weeks gestation to 6 weeks of age.

    b. birth to 4 weeks of age.

    c. birth to 6 months of age.

    d. 1 month to 12 months of age.

3. Illness or disability may interfere with the process of growth and development in children. T. Berry Brazelton describes critical periods of development as

    a. developmental landmarks.

    b. touch points.

    c. developmental stages.

    d. foundational milestones.

4. An individual is exhibiting which of Kohlberg's Stages of Moral Development when he or she feels "duty bound" to maintain social order?

    a. Preconventional

    b. Formal operations

    c. Conventional

    d. Moralistic consciousness

5. According to Erikson's stages of psychosocial development, which of the following stages of development would a person be in if the task to be achieved is to view one's life as meaningful and fulfilling?

    a. Identity vs. role diffusion

    b. Intimacy vs. isolation

    c. Generativity vs. stagnation

    d. Integrity vs. despair

6. Match the age of embryonic development with the developmental characteristic.

    _____ week 4   a. Maturation of the respiratory system

    _____ week 6   b. Fetal movement felt by mother

    _____ week 20   c. Limb bud distinguishable

    _____ week 28   d. Heart structure and circulatory pathway established

    _____ week 32   e. Lanugo present

Labeling Exercise

7. What reflex is the infant exhibiting in this photograph?

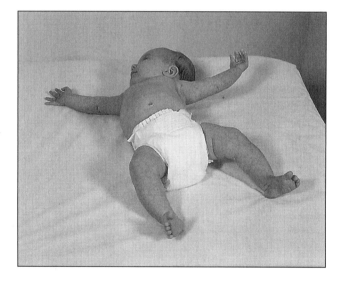

_____

8. A major psychological task of neonates is to _____ with parents.

9. In which stage of Piaget's phases of cognitive development is the ability to see relationships and to do abstract thinking developed?

    a. Sensorimotor

    b. Preoperational

    c. Concrete operations

    d. Formal operations

10. At what age would you expect a child to form short, simple sentences?

    a. 1 year

    b. 18 months

    c. 2 years

    d. 3 years

11. Place the following stages of faith, according to Fowler, in the proper sequence.

    _____ Conjunctive faith

    _____ Universalizing faith

    _____ Intuitive-projective faith

    _____ Mythical-literal faith

    _____ Undifferentiated faith

    _____ Individuative-reflective faith

    _____ Synthetic-conventional faith

12. Immediately following delivery, the nurse performs an assessment of the infant and assigns an Apgar score. Which signs does the nurse observe?

    a. Muscle tone, sucking ability, skin color, and presence of meconium

    b. Heart rate, respiratory rate, blood pressure, and body temperature

    c. Reflex irritability, crying, grasp, and muscle tone

    d. Heart rate, color, respiratory effort, muscle tone, and reflex irritability

13. Which of the following is the leading cause of death in young children?

    a. Suicide

    b. Respiratory disease

    c. Sports injuries

    d. Accidents

14. When teaching a preadolescent female about menstrual periods, which of the following statements would be accurate to relate?

    a. The average age of menarche is 10 years old.

    b. The menstrual cycle becomes regular after about 6 to 12 months.

    c. Many American females experience premenstrual syndrome.

    d. During the first few menstrual cycles, females do not ovulate.

15. The nurse is evaluating the developmental level of a 2-year-old. Which characteristics should the nurse expect to observe in this age child?

    a. The toddler interacts well with other children and shares toys.

    b. The toddler is able to tie shoelaces and dress herself.

    c. The toddler should weigh four times more than birth weight.

    d. The toddler knows the difference between past and present.

16. Recommended health screening for adolescents includes

    a. asking about school performance, and alcohol and tobacco use.

    b. discussing sexual activity and assessing for eating disorders.

    c. performing body mass measurement and cholesterol testing.

    d. administering hepatitis B vaccine and HIV testing if indicated.

    e. All of the above may be appropriate as adolescent screening measurements.

Critical Thinking

17. A mother of a toddler expresses her concerns that her child is a "picky" eater. She asks the nurse what she should do to get her toddler to eat. What response should the nurse give to this mother? What other information does she need to obtain before offering advice?

1. Which factors are considered the most important predicators of illness in young adults?

    a. Complications related to chronic health problems

    b. Latent effects of genetic defects

    c. Stress and ineffective coping mechanisms

    d. Issues of social isolation

2. Nursing interventions designed to assist the young adult to successfully manage the physiological challenge of transitioning between adolescence and adulthood include

    a. encouraging socialization.

    b. encouraging the development of a healthy lifestyle.

    c. identifying appropriate retirement strategies.

    d. assessing the client's belief systems.

3. According to Erickson's stages of psychosocial development, which stage would a person be in if the task to be achieved is to reflect on the past and anticipate the future?

    a. Integrity vs. despair

    b. Intimacy vs. isolation

    c. Generativity vs. stagnation

    d. Identity vs. role diffusion

4. According to Havighurst's theory of psychosocial development, which major life event in the middle adult years is linked to feelings of depression or happiness?

    a. The return of adult children to the home

    b. Early retirement

    c. The empty nest syndrome

    d. The death of a parent

5. A health promotion intervention strategy appropriate for a group of 20-year-olds would be

   a. teaching a self-breast examination class to men and women.

   b. developing a program to screen for hearing loss.

   c. holding a health fair at a local supermarket.

   d. promoting independence by supporting legislation for fair housing.

6. A personality characteristic of generally healthy individuals who view life as a challenge and not a problem is _____.

7. Match the stage of psychosocial development in the left column with its associated developmental phase in the right column.

   _____ feels good about oneself and   a. Young adult
           achievements

   _____ believes will always   b. Middle adult
           belong to parents

   _____ has increased concerns about   c. Young adult transition
           stress and work

   _____ develops a sense of civic awareness

   _____ experiences changing family roles

8. The nurse is preparing a 25-year-old college student for an outpatient procedure. After the teaching session, the client expresses feelings of anxiety. The client will benefit most if he receives emotional support from whom?

   a. Friends

   b. Parents

   c. Older sister

   d. Teacher

9. If the nurse believes that psychosocial stresses are impairing a 45-year-old client's ability to cope with a minor illness, the nurse needs to asses the client's

   a. problem-solving abilities.

   b. home and work relationships.

   c. pain indicators.

   d. spiritual belief systems.

10. A 49-year-old client has launched her last child and decides to return to work and school. She tells you she is also getting ready to have a make-over and change her hairstyle. This client is most likely experiencing

    a. empty nest syndrome.

    b. midlife crises.

    c. menopause.

    d. role reversal.

11. A 52-year-old client is worried about his health. He is the same age as his wife, who has been diagnosed with hypertension. What advice is appropriate for health promotion and disease prevention at this time in his life?

    a. Decrease activity but maintain caloric intake to keep weight steady and prevent stress-induced illnesses.

    b. Schedule an eye exam every 3 to 5 years for glaucoma and macular degeneration.

    c. Continue regular, yearly physical exams, including prostate and breast exams.

    d. Maintain steady diet and activity, and schedule physical exams every 3 to 5 years.

12. Which educational intervention would be appropriate for a middle-aged adult regarding physiological changes?

    a. Instruct men that enlargement of the prostate gland is common.

    b. Encourage a balance of exercise/activity, rest, and sleep.

    c. Instruct about fall precautions.

    d. Teach about the need for adequate calcium intake as part of a balanced diet.

13. Which topic would the nurse develop as a focus of a wellness program for a group of middle-aged adults?

    a. Stress management

    b. Home safety

    c. Suicide prevention

    d. Increased socialization

Critical Thinking

14. A client presents to the clinic with nonspecific somatic complaints. He reports feeling stressed out and unsure about his life's work and all of the many changes in his life. He tells the nurse, "I am just too young to be a grandfather." What is the likely stage of growth and development the client is experiencing? Identify nursing strategies appropriate to assisting the client with successful transition through this stage of development.

1. By 2030 adults over age 65 are projected to make up what percentage of the total U.S. population?

   a. 5%

   b. 11%

   c. 16%

   d. 20%

2. Which of the following is the greatest problem in the homebound elderly?

   a. Malnutrition

   b. Falls

   c. Uncontrolled diabetes

   d. Loneliness

3. An expectation of the older adult in this stage of growth and development is to accept one's life as it is. Which of the following actions would facilitate this goal?

   a. Encourage the use of reminiscence.

   b. Assess for body image changes.

   c. Instruct about the benefits of proper nutrition and exercise.

   d. Encourage socialization.

4. The hearing loss associated with old age is called

   a. presbycusis.

   b. presbyopia.

   c. presbycardia.

   d. otitis media.

5. Match the pathologic visual change experienced by the elderly in the left column with its description from the right column.

_____ macular degeneration   a. Opacity of the lens of the eye

_____ cataracts   b. Inability of the lens to accommodate for near vision

_____ glaucoma   c. Increased intraocular pressure

_____ presbyopia   d. Loss of central vision

6. Which of the following physiological changes, associated with aging, would support the need to teach a preoperative 78-year-old client deep breathing, coughing, and incentive spirometry exercises?

a. Fewer functioning alveoli and decrease in the number of cilia

b. Decrease in peristaltic activity

c. Slowed transmission of nerve impulses

d. The development of lentigo senilis

7. Aging is associated with altered functioning of the pancreas. Which of the following would a nurse evaluate in order to assess this problem?

a. Blood glucose level

b. Blood urea nitrogen level

c. Bowel sounds

d. Blood potassium level

8. Which statement indicates an understanding by the nurse of hearing loss as it occurs in the older adult?

a. "Older adults are easily distracted by external stimuli."

b. "Older adults respond to high- and low-pitched sounds about equally."

c. "Older adults and teens are likely to experience the same rate of hearing loss."

d. "Older adults respond best to low-pitched sounds."

9. Which nursing intervention may help calm an agitated client who has been diagnosed with dementia?

a. Turn out overhead lights.

b. Offer support by gently touching the client.

c. Turn on soft music to distract the client.

d. Encourage participation in a group activity.

10. Which of the following statements is true regarding wound healing in the elderly? Wounds heal

    a. at the same rate as in middle-aged adults.

    b. faster than in middle-aged adults.

    c. slower than in middle-aged adults.

11. Which of the following strategies would be appropriate to teach an elderly client regarding skin care?

    a. Avoid tub baths.

    b. Use tepid water during baths.

    c. Rub the skin briskly while drying the skin.

    d. Use alcohol to soothe itchy dry skin areas.

12. Mrs. Carpenter, 82 years old, was admitted to your unit yesterday with pneumonia. She is running a consistent low-grade fever, is dehydrated, and has difficulty getting out of bed due to stiffness in her right hip and knee joints. Her mental examination results in the following findings: she is disoriented, with the disorientation worsening at night; she mumbles incoherently at times; she has difficulty concentrating on simple tasks such as feeding herself; and she calls out in fear to the nurses to remove the bugs that are crawling up the privacy curtain in her room. Her son states that she was not this way at home, that she was alert and oriented. Which of the following best summarizes the clinical features of Mrs. Carpenter's mental status? She is

    a. acutely confused.

    b. suffering from dementia.

    c. experiencing an episode of depression.

    d. suffering from a personality disorder.

13. Which statement best describes the nurse's understanding of the use of reminiscence therapy as an intervention when caring for an older client?

    a. "It is used to raise the client's self-esteem."

    b. "It is used to put one's life in perspective."

    c. "It is used successfully with agitated clients."

    d. "It is best used in a group setting."

14. Match the age-related change in the left column with its impact on drug therapy from the right column.

_____ less total body fluid

_____ increased adipose tissue

_____ reduced liver size and decreased hepatic metabolism

_____ reduction in glomerular filtration rate, decrease in number of nephrons

_____ drier oral mucosa

_____ less muscle mass

_____ reduced circulation to lower bowel and vagina

a. Difficulty absorbing usual intramuscular adult dose at a single injection site

b. Higher level of water-soluble drugs

c. Greater accumulation of fat-soluble drugs

d. Slower metabolism and longer half-life of some drugs

e. Prolonged melting times for suppositories

f. Difficulty swallowing tablets and capsules

g. Slower elimination of some drugs

15. When taking a medication history of an elderly client, which of the following should be assessed in addition to the client's prescription drugs?

a. Potential interactions with foods

b. Use of over-the-counter medications

c. How medications are obtained

d. All of the above

16. Which of the following types of elder abuse is imposed social isolation?

a. Psychological abuse

b. Physical abuse

c. Neglect

d. Exploitation

17. Mrs. Freidman was admitted to your long-term care facility today. Which of the following interventions would promote her safety during her stay?

a. Teach her about correct medication administration.

b. Orient her to her surroundings.

c. Provide large-print materials for her to read.

d. Help her to focus on her abilities instead of her limitations.

Critical Thinking

18. A 75-year-old client tells the nurse that several of her friends have fallen and have had to have hip replacement surgery. She tells the nurse she just doesn't understand how this is happening because they are all so careful. She confides that she is afraid she will also need hip replacement surgery. What are factors that contribute to falls in the older adult? What interventions are appropriate in this situation?

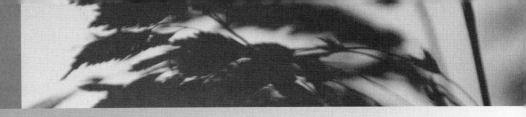

CHAPTER 20   Acute Care

1. *Acute care* is defined as

    a. rehabilitative care in an extended-care facility.

    b. short-term hospital care with fewer than 30 days' length of stay.

    c. outpatient treatment occurring within a 23-hour time frame.

    d. wellness preventive care administered in a medical screening clinic.

2. Hepatitis B vaccine series administered to nursing students prior to their beginning work in the clinical area is an example of

    a. primary prevention.

    b. secondary prevention.

    c. tertiary prevention.

    d. chronic disease prevention.

3. Facilities that are designed to care for critically ill clients with multisystem disorders who require on average 25 days of care are referred to as _____.

4. List the four general categories of advanced practice nurses.

    a. _____

    b. _____

    c. _____

    d. _____

5. Cite the three factors identified by expert nurses that are requisite for clinical decision making.

    a. _____

    b. _____

    c. _____

6. Which is an example of an acute care unit in which clients with common problems are matched with specially trained staff?

    a. Neonatal intensive care unit

    b. Cardiac surgical intensive care unit

    c. Neurological intensive care unit

    d. All of the above

7. Information that is systematically developed to assist health care practitioners in clinical practice situations is referred to as

    a. the nursing process.

    b. quality indicators.

    c. clinical guidelines.

    d. best practice.

8. Care maps or clinical pathways

    a. can only be used by the registered nurse in planning care.

    b. help reduce variations in care and resource utilization.

    c. are only developed for acute-care interventions.

    d. improve client outcomes but prolong hospitalization.

9. The federal agency that provides health care professionals with evidence-based clinical practice guidelines and related documents is

    a. the Cochrane Collaboration.

    b. the Robert Wood Johnson Foundation.

    c. the Centers for Disease Control.

    d. the Agency for Healthcare Research and Quality.

10. The mission of the Joint Commission on Accreditation of Healthcare Organizations is to

    a. protect the health of American workers.

    b. promote health and quality of life by preventing and controlling disease, injury, and disability.

    c. continuously improve the safety and quality of care provided to the public.

    d. advance and disseminate scientific knowledge to improve human health.

11. The largest health care system in the United States is

    a. Kaiser Permanente.

    b. the American Hospital Association.

    c. the Veterans Health Administration of the Department of Veterans Affairs.

    d. the Johns Hopkins Medical System.

12. List three social issues that impact acute care nursing.

    a. _____

    b. _____

    c. _____

13. The issue of entry into practice relates to

    a. the practice of delegating nursing duties to unlicensed personnel.

    b. the point at which stressors overwhelm a client and require acute-care nursing intervention.

    c. the period in which a nurse is considered a novice practitioner.

    d. the minimal education preparation to become a registered nurse.

14. *The St. Joseph's Hospital E.D. Diagnostic and Treatment Process for Thrombolytic Therapy for Stroke Patients* guides the health care practitioner in whether or not a patient may be a candidate for thrombolytic therapy with tPA. What is a major temporal criterion for treatment with thrombolytic drugs?

    _____

Critical Thinking

15. Discuss what the term *evidence-based practice* means and how this concept will change the art and practice of nursing.

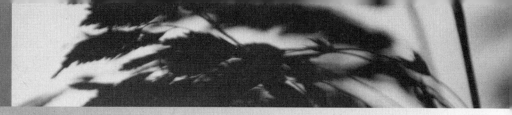

1. The focus of restorative care is on

   a. curing the client.

   b. assisting the client to the highest level of functioning.

   c. keeping the client dependent on health care providers.

   d. ensuring that a client regains his or her pre-illness heath state.

2. The process in which a person is aided in achieving optimum physical, emotional, psychosocial, and vocational potential is called

   a. hospice care.

   b. developmental balance.

   c. rehabilitation.

   d. life balance.

3. Which legislation has a major impact on changing the philosophy of long-term care from custodial to restorative?

   a. The Omnibus Budget Act of 1978

   b. The Health Insurance Portability and Accountability Act of 1996

   c. The Elder Justice Act of 2003

   d. The Social Security Act of 1935

4. The Americans with Disabilities Act of 1990

   a. barred guide dogs from public places.

   b. ordered that employers hire a disabled person in place of a nondisabled person.

   c. mandated that all physical barriers be removed in areas of work, transportation, and education.

   d. required that nursing home residents not be physically restrained.

5. The World Health Organization defines disability as

    a. loss of function at the organ level.

    b. inability to perform life roles due to disability.

    c. functional limitation in ability to perform activities of daily living.

    d. restriction or lack of ability to perform an activity a normal person can perform.

6. Which is an example of restorative care that may begun by nurses in the acute-care setting?

    a. Range of motion exercises

    b. Management of acute pain

    c. Chest tube drainage monitoring

    d. Intracranial pressure measurement

7. The typical length of stay in a subacute facility is

    a. 2 to 5 days.

    b. 7 to 9 days.

    c. 10 to 14 days.

    d. 14 to 21 days.

8. Restorative care is provided across the lifespan. Which group would require cardiac rehabilitative restorative nursing care?

    a. Children

    b. Adolescents

    c. Young adults

    d. Late middle-aged adults

9. List two physiological conditions associated with aging that may complicate or prolong restorative care.

    a. _____

    b. _____

10. Acuity describes

    a. the developmental age of the client.

    b. the degree of dependence or independence the client demonstrates.

    c. the total amount of acute-care nursing hours that a client requires.

    d. the method of reimbursement for rehabilitative services.

11. Frequent comorbidities among the elderly include

   a. AIDS, stroke, and heart failure.

   b. cystic fibrosis, renal failure, and diabetes.

   c. myocardial infarction, cancer, and anemia.

   d. chronic obstructive pulmonary disease and Alzheimer's.

12. The Joint Commission on Accreditation of Healthcare Organizations (JCAHO) recommends that an interdisciplinary team consist of six professionals. Which disciplines do they represent?

   a. _____

   b. _____

   c. _____

   d. _____

   e. _____

   f. _____

13. Match the health team member in the left column with their role in the right column.

   _____ occupational therapist   a. Swallow evaluation

   _____ vocational counselor   b. Case management

   _____ clinical nurse specialist   c. Self-care skills

   _____ speech therapist   d. Adaptation of work setting

14. Which nursing theorist developed a model of self-care?

   a. Virginia Henderson

   b. Sr. Callista Roy

   c. Dorothea Orem

   b. Hildegarde Peplau

15. An elderly woman, who is the sole provider of care for her chronically ill spouse, complains of not getting enough rest and of feeling fatigued. Which nursing diagnosis would the nurse select in planning care for this woman?

   a. Impaired physical mobility

   b. Self-care deficit

   c. Spiritual distress

   d. Caregiver role strain

Critical Thinking

16. An 82-year-old male who suffered a stroke is a candidate for restorative care. His son has never heard of this type of care and asks you if his father is being sent to a nursing home, where he'll get a bedsore and die. How would you respond to the son's question?

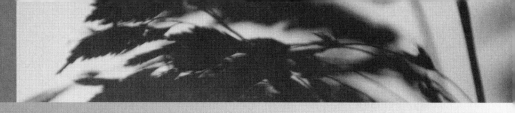

1. Which statement best describes the impact of Medicare on home health nursing?

    a. There has been no significant change on the focus of care.

    b. The focus of care has shifted from mother-child care to care of the frail elderly.

    c. Nursing care in the home remains focused on health promotion and disease prevention activities.

    d. Private insurers no longer cover direct-care nursing services.

2. Identify the three credentials a home care agency must have to demonstrate compliance with standards.

    a. _____

    b. _____

    c. _____

3. In order to maintain Medicare certification, a home care agency must

    a. be periodically evaluated by an external accrediting body.

    b. receive approval by the American Nurses Association.

    c. offer services to indigent people.

    d. be licensed by multiple third-party payers.

4. Which statement best describes home health care nursing as practiced in today's health care environment?

    a. Nursing care provided to acutely ill elderly who are homebound.

    b. Multidisciplinary array of services to clients who meet insurance requirements.

    c. The primary goal is health restoration and promotion.

    d. It does not require a special body of knowledge.

5. Home health care nursing requires that nurses

   a. apply all aspects of the nursing process.

   b. balance clients' rights with government regulations.

   c. obtain a written contract before beginning care.

   d. practice the three levels of prevention only if reimbursed by insurers.

6. The legislation that set forth the rules determining who could receive care and the payment system for that care is specified under Medicare

   a. Parts A and B.

   b. Conditions of Participation.

   c. Social Security Act of 1965, Title IX.

   d. Prospective Payment System.

7. List the characteristics that distinguish home health nursing care from home hospice nursing care.

   _____

8. Proprietary home care agencies include

   a. public health departments.

   b. nonprofit home care organizations.

   c. private, for-profit organizations.

   d. voluntary agencies.

9. The home care nurse is visiting an elderly client to assess wound status post surgery. She determines that the client is able to change the dressing but does not understand why it should be changed every day. Based on the assessment data given, the nursing diagnosis for this client is

   a. deficient knowledge.

   b. ineffective coping.

   c. alteration in skin integrity.

   d. ineffective therapeutic regimen.

10. The long-term goal of the home care nurse for any client regardless of diagnosis is to

   a. develop a network of support systems for the client and family.

   b. promote independent functioning.

   c. change the client's lifestyle practices.

   d. manage and evaluate the client care plan.

11. Home health care services under the Medicare guidelines require the nurse to provide _____ care to eligible clients.

   a. daily, short-term

   b. intermittent, long-term

   c. intermittent, short-term

   d. at least hourly

12. Which of the following is considered skilled care under the Medicare guidelines?

   a. Hospice home care

   b. Management and evaluation of a care plan

   c. Chronic care management

   d. Respite care

13. The nurse makes a home visit to a client who has not been checking daily blood glucose levels. The client tells the nurse that someone else is going to have to do it, maybe the home health aide. Which action should the nurse take first?

   a. Call the home health supervisor to find an aide who knows how to use a glucometer.

   b. Assess the client's clinical status, both physical and emotional.

   c. Call the physician and report the client as noncompliant with therapeutic regimen.

   d. Document the client's noncompliance.

14. The home care nurse is making an initial visit to a homebound elderly client. When she arrives at the home she observes there are several bars on the block and a group of men hanging on the corner playing cards. What action should the nurse take?

   a. Park as close to the client's home as possible and go in quickly.

   b. Return to the agency and request an escort to go with her into the neighborhood.

   c. Call the client on her cell phone and reschedule the visit for another day.

   d. Call the police and report suspicion of illegal behavior.

Critical Thinking

15. The home health nurse is developing a plan of care for a 72-year-old client, newly diagnosed with insulin-dependent diabetes mellitus. The client's family members express anxiety about the client's ability to function after discharge from home care. They tell the nurse the client has paid into Medicare and deserves to have someone come to the home for as long as possible. How would the nurse handle this situation?

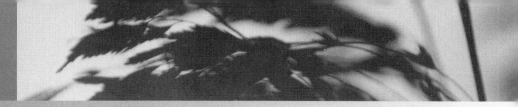

1. A group of people who share common characteristics and/or geographic location is referred to as a

   a. special-interest group.

   b. community.

   c. neighborhood.

   d. aggregate.

2. Which question(s) would provide the nurse with information to assist in development of realistic health goals for the community?

   a. "How does the community conform to regional laws?"

   b. "Do you have a community association?"

   c. "Tell me how the community defines itself and its purpose?"

   d. "How well does the community relate to its neighbors?"

3. The nurse who uses critical social theory to drive nursing care is interested in promoting what?

   a. Self-efficacy of the community

   b. Social change to enhance the health of the community

   c. Environmental justice

   d. Nursing's agenda for health care reform

4. Match the level of community participation in the left column with the appropriate description in the right column.

   _____ informing   a. Negotiation between citizens and power holders

   _____ consultation   b. Citizen's power assures accountability of program

   _____ partnership   c. One-way flow of information

   _____ delegated power   d. Participants have full governance of medical decisions

   _____ citizen control   e. Get citizen views, no guarantee to use those views

5. The primary responsibility of community health nurses is to

    a. ensure access to essential health care services for families.

    b. promote the functional independence and wellness of all members.

    c. advocate for safe housing and neighborhood clinics.

    d. provide educational programs to at-risk population groups.

6. A community health nurse teaches a group of teenagers the dangers of using club drugs. What role is the nurse assuming?

    a. Facilitator

    b. Advocate

    c. Educator

    d. Counselor

7. The Lauraville community association has gathered data about West Nile virus, established an information hotline, and developed a program to educate members about the issue. This is an example of

    a. delegation of power.

    b. citizen control.

    c. informing.

    d. educating.

8. Direct care is considered the purview of community health nurses. Identify at least two of the environments in which direct care occurs.

    a. _____

    b. _____

9. A teacher contacts the school nurse and requests that a case conference be set for the parents of a disabled child. This situation is an example of

    a. case finding.

    b. collaboration.

    c. counseling.

    d. advocacy.

10. The community health nurse makes a visit to the home of a pregnant teenager who has not kept her prenatal appointments. The teen reports she does not have money for transportation and does not know how to get to the clinic. An expected outcome of the visit is

   a. the client will attend all future prenatal visits.

   b. the client will describe resources available for assistance with transportation.

   c. the client will access all available resources.

   d. the client will report successful delivery.

11. The community is concerned about the increased numbers of teenagers hospitalized for drug- and alcohol-related incidents and asks the community health nurse to implement an educational awareness program. How should the nurse proceed?

   a. Consult with MADD to develop new advertising campaigns that include the dangers of drug use leading to hospitalization.

   b. Analyze city and hospital statistics to identify the nature and extent of the problem.

   c. Meet with local legislators to advocate for an increase in the legal age at which one can purchase alcohol.

   d. Consult all area middle and high schools to determine whether the school nurses believe the problem requires immediate attention.

12. Which of the following is the responsibility of school health nurses?

   a. Making periodic visits to each child's home

   b. Designing educational programs to meet the needs of disabled children

   c. Identifying high-risk children and making proper referrals

   d. Planning and coordinating after-school activities

13. Health care priorities based on Healthy People 2010 objectives include

   a. provision of adequate services to the chronically ill elderly.

   b. health prevention and primary care services.

   c. initiatives to fund more family nurse practitioners.

   d. increasing services to correctional facilities.

14. The first issue for nurses to consider when working with communities is that of acceptance by the community. Which action would be most likely to foster acceptance?

    a. Participate in community activities and establish rapport with members.

    b. Arrange an introduction by the head of the community organization.

    c. Offer to contribute a large sum of money to the organization's fund-raising event.

    d. Establish a scholarship for the local high school.

Critical Thinking

15. The community health nurse is asked to assist the community in developing a safe neighbors program. What approach should the nurse take? What roles will be employed by the nurse?

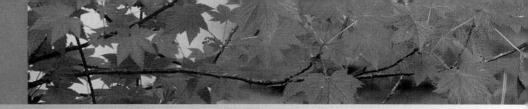

1. Defining characteristics of the "great man" theory of leadership suggests that

    a. leadership ability is based on one's ability to engage with others.

    b. some people are born great leaders and innately know how to lead.

    c. all people have the potential to become great leaders.

    d. knowledge of the intimate details of a situation makes one a great leader.

2. _____ describes a belief that leadership is based on the needs of others and on helping others become healthy, wise, and autonomous.

3. According to the leadership hierarchy theory, nurses function best at the highest level.

    a. What is the defining characteristic of this level? _____

    b. Why is this style considered a "best fit" for nurses? _____

4. The nurse manager describes her leadership style as transformational. It is expected that she

    a. works best with those who like and need direction.

    b. uses inspiration, motivation, and vision to empower her staff.

    c. is controlling in her approach to guiding others.

    d. demonstrates limited flexibility when others approach with new ideas.

5. A nurse on your unit describes the charge nurse as being "all about power. She gets things done but doesn't seem to have a vision for what can be accomplished," the nurse tells you. What does this suggest about the charge nurse's leadership style?

    _____

6. A conflict has developed among several staff members over the use of the break room on the unit. The nurse manager, using a democratic leadership style, will deal with the issue by

   a. calling a meeting and asking staff members for their input on resolving the problem.

   b. asking the nursing supervisor to intervene on her behalf.

   c. waiting to see whether the staff will resolve the problem without intervention.

   d. closing the break room and instructing the staff the best thing for the unit would be for everyone to go off-unit for breaks.

7. Which statement best describes an autocratic approach to leading?

   a. "Let's get everyone together to discuss the situation and decide on a plan of action as a group."

   b. "Just send in your reports and I will develop the plan of action needed to resolve the problem."

   c. "Come to the meeting and you will have an opportunity to ask questions before the plan of action is implemented."

   d. "Next meeting we will develop teams to work on the problem, and each team will present a plan of action."

8. A colleague reports she has been appointed head of a committee to develop new guidelines for infection control. When asked about her plan for getting the tasks accomplished, she tells you she is not worried about a plan—"It will get done." This is an example of which style of leading?

   a. Autocratic

   b. Consultative

   c. Participative

   d. Laissez-faire

9. Which statement best reflects the prevailing attitude about how people develop leadership skills?

   a. A leadership role requires a person to be prepared to apply known knowledge and learn new approaches.

   b. Skills are developed primarily through gaining theoretical knowledge and not necessarily through practice.

   c. Observing a good mentor is sufficient for developing leadership skills.

   d. Leaders are born not made.

10. In order to be an effective leader and member of a multidisciplinary team _____ is essential skill for all nurses.

    a. advocacy

    b. collaboration

    c. partnering

    d. delegating

11. Match the type of leadership style in the left column with an example of it from the right column.

    _____ autocratic

    _____ democratic

    _____ consultative

    _____ laissez-faire

    _____ situational

    a. The unit manager allows an aggressive staff member to consistently dominate the staff meetings.

    b. The leader of the risk management committee is directive at times, while at other times lets the group problem-solve.

    c. The case manager gives background information about the client's case to the multidisciplinary team, and then invites discussion about the client's plan of care.

    d. The unit manager tells the staff what will be done to solve the unit's staffing problem.

    e. The unit manager encourages everyone to ask questions and seek understanding of the issues.

12. In which of the following styles of leadership would the expected outcome be the empowerment of group members?

    a. Autocratic

    b. Democratic

    c. Laissez-faire

    d. Situational

13. The UAP assigned to your unit approaches you and asks if she can change the dressing around your cltient's G-tube. Which of the following questions would you *first* answer in order to make a decision whether to delegate this task to the UAP?

    a. "Is the UAP competent to do the task?"

    b. "Can this task be delegated?"

    c. "If I delegate this task, will it put my client at risk?"

    d. "What do the physician's orders say about this?"

14. The nurse manager is developing a budget for the next fiscal year. She asks you to attend a meeting with housekeeping department and report on the status of any new hires or layoffs in that department. The manager is gathering information related to _____.

15. Which of the following reflects positive mentor behavior?

    a. An experienced staff nurse readily offers the answer to any questions.

    b. A unit manager allows a novice nurse to find a solution to a clinical problem.

    c. The chairperson of a newly formed committee allows the committee members to find their own direction.

    d. A nursing instructor offers to coach a nursing student in exchange for babysitting services.

16. Identify three critical elements of self-awareness.

    a. _____

    b. _____

    c. _____

17. Delegation is an essential skill for an effective leader. Effective delegation requires the nurse manager to

    a. get permission from the employee before assigning tasks, especially odious ones.

    b. allow freedom of choice in assignments to ensure high morale on the unit.

    c. know what tasks can be safely delegated to whom and to communicate the assignment in measurable terms.

    d. be directive in her approach, seeking commitment from but not permission of the employee.

Critical Thinking

18. The unit has just hired a new nurse manager. The previous manager was an authoritative leader; the new manager has a democratic style of leading. What impact will this have on the functioning of the unit? What recommendations can you as a staff nurse make to support the manager as she transitions to her role?

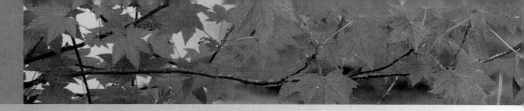

1. Match the terms on the left with the appropriate definition on the right.

    _____ quality assurance
    _____ quality domains
    _____ dimensions of quality performance
    _____ quality
    _____ continuous quality
    _____ total quality management

    a. Meeting or exceeding requirements of the customer
    b. Structure, process, and outcome
    c. A method of management that views the employee as a resource
    d. Problem solving to work toward quality care
    e. The scientific approach used to study work processes improvement
    f. Efficacy, appropriateness, availability, timeliness, effectiveness, continuity, safety, efficiency, respect, and caring

2. Medical errors are a significant cause of death and injury in the United States. To minimize these occurrences, it is recommended that

    a. individuals be held accountable for these errors.
    b. work-flow enhancements are put into place.
    c. system errors are corrected.

3. During a team meeting, the unit manager reports that the clients are increasingly complaining that their call lights are not being answered in a timely fashion. Staff nurse Smith says to her coworker, staff nurse Jennings, "There is nothing we can do about it. We are so short-staffed." Nurse Jennings, who knows that quality improvement is a team responsibility, says

    a. "We could really use extra help, but it is up to the hospital administration to let us hire more staff."
    b. "I'm sure we can manage if we all pitch in."
    c. "We should all meet to study the problem together and develop some solutions."
    d. "Don't look at me, I answer my clients' call lights as soon as I can."

4. The _____ is accountable for performance improvement.

    a. facility director

    b. individual employee

    c. unit manager

    d. customer

5. Failure of a health care facility to adhere to federally mandated health care standards can result in which of the following actions?

    a. The chief operating officer can be arrested.

    b. Employees can be dismissed at will.

    c. Federal funding and payment can be denied.

    d. The facility can be shut down.

6. Which of the following federal regulations established denial of payment for substandard care?

    a. Consolidated Omnibus Budget Reconciliation Act

    b. Social Security Act

    c. Omnibus Budget Reconciliation Act

    d. Patient Self-Determination Act

7. A staff nurse in a hospital is responsible for providing direct care to clients and considers a client as a customer. To what other "customers" is the nurse accountable within the hospital?

    _____

    _____

8. Standards of care, algorithms, procedures, and guidelines are developed by health care organizations to

    a. be used as a framework to ensure delivery of quality health care and reduce liability.

    b. ensure that client advocacy is a primary nursing role.

    c. prevent individual health care providers from establishing policies regarding client care.

    d. establish credibility for any activity not sanctioned by JCAHO requirements.

9. Which of the following organizational characteristics would you expect to find in a high-performance organization?

   a. The organization operates hierarchically.

   b. Conflict is welcome and considered helpful.

   c. The atmosphere is political.

   d. The staff are the authority on care of the client.

10. List three characteristics of quality nursing care.

   a. _____

   b. _____

   c. _____

11. In a unit meeting, the unit manager reported that the readmission rate of surgical clients had increased. The primary reason for readmission was wound infection. In this situation, which of the following health care providers carries the responsibility for quality improvement?

   a. The nurses

   b. The physicians

   c. The unlicensed assistive personnel

   d. All health care providers

12. What term refers to the collection of data from client records and the subsequent comparison of this data to a set of predetermined criteria? _____

13. "Nurses are expected to know the policies and procedures of the organization and to keep hallways free of clutter and equipment." This meets which environment of care standard?

   a. Security management

   b. Utilities management

   c. Fire prevention

   d. Emergency management

14. _____, _____, and _____ are activities nurses engage in that will have an impact on the policy-making process.

15. Algorithms used by nurses in health care organizations are best described as

    a. a specific set of step-by-step directions about how a nurse is to perform a procedure or conduct an activity.

    b. guidelines that describe best practice standards.

    c. a tool delineating the extent and character of the nurse's duty to a client.

    d. graphical representation depicting a set of steps the nurse uses in a particular clinical situation to guide decision-making process.

Critical Thinking

16. Your organization has failed to receive accreditation from JCAHO. The nurse manager reports supplemental recommendations were made that must be remedied. A new nurse questions the findings and asks what happened. She is worried and is considering leaving the organization. How would the nurse manager handle this?

1. Regulated medical waste includes

   a. all waste generated in a health care setting.

   b. only used needles, syringes, and sharp objects.

   c. unconsumed food remaining on the client's food tray.

   d. dressings saturated with serosanguineous drainage and bodily fluid specimens.

2. The Centers for Disease Control (CDC) recommends that health care professionals

   a. use standard precautions only with infectious clients.

   b. adopt transmission-based precautions when caring for all clients.

   c. wear a N95 respirator when caring for clients with tuberculosis.

   d. don a surgical face mask when caring for clients on airborne precautions.

3. Match the term in the left column with its explanation in the right column.

   _____ virulence   a. The place for the organism to live

   _____ colonization   b. The degree of pathogenicity of an infection's microorganism

   _____ reservoir   c. An entity that is capable of causing disease

   _____ agent   d. Multiplication of microorganisms on or within a host that does not result in cellular injury

4. The procedure of surgical handwashing differs from ordinary handwashing in which way?

   a. The hands and forearms are held above elbow level while rinsing with water.

   b. The hands and forearms are dried in the direction of most clean to least clean.

   c. Warm water and friction are used only with the surgical handwashing procedure.

   d. There are no differences in procedure technique.

5. In the home setting, boiling objects renders them clean, not sterile. With this in mind, how long would the nurse advise the client to boil an object and at what temperature?

   _____

6. A nurse cleaning a used surgical instrument rinses blood and bodily fluid from the object with cold water. What is the rationale for using cold water?

_____

7. A 4-year-old child requires droplet precautions for the chickenpox virus. How will the nurse who is caring for this child best approach the situation?

    a. Allow the child to play with a cap and mask to promote comfort.

    b. Show the child his or her face from the doorway before putting a mask on.

    c. Encourage the child to dress a favorite stuffed animal or doll with a cap and mask.

    d. All of the above examples are appropriate for a child in a restricted setting.

8. Which set of factors increases a client's susceptibility for infection?

    a. Advanced age and comorbid conditions

    b. Immunosuppression following chemotherapy treatment

    c. Inadequate protein intake and poor skin integrity

    d. All of these conditions increase a client's susceptibility for infection

9. Name two nursing interventions that will help to decrease pathogen transmission.

    a. _____

    b. _____

10. A client is admitted with dehydration secondary to diarrhea. Which infection control measure should the nurse use? (You may select more than one.)

    a. Place the newly admitted client with another client who is also having diarrhea.

    b. Obtain a private room and use standard precautions.

    c. Place the client in a negative airflow room and adopt contact precautions.

    d. Wear a nonsterile gown if soiling of uniform is likely.

11. Which vaccine does the federal agency OSHA require that health care agencies make available to their employees?

    a. Meningococcal vaccine

    b. *Haemophilus influenzae* vaccine

    c. Pneumococcal vaccine

    d. Hepatitis B vaccine

12. A visitor asks what he may bring as a gift to a hospitalized immunosuppressd client. The nurse suggests that he bring a

    a. fresh fruit basket.

    b. compact disc and player for listening enjoyment.

    c. puppy to keep the client company.

    d. geranium in a clay pot.

13. When a child is immunized against varicella, the child receives

    a. passive immunity.

    b. active immunity.

    c. acquired immunity.

    d. artificial immunity.

14. The cells that produce antibodies in response to antigens are called

    a. natural killer cells.

    b. neutrophils.

    c. plasma cells.

    d. helper T cells.

15. The time interval from the onset of nonspecific symptoms until specific symptoms of the infectious process begin to manifest is called the

    a. illness stage.

    b. convalescent stage.

    c. incubation period.

    d. prodromal stage.

Critical Thinking

16. The nurse who is handling new admissions to a medical-surgical unit is expecting four clients but has only one private room available. Which of the following clients should be assigned to a private room? Discuss your decision-making process and how you assigned priority to this individual.

    Client 1: A client admitted for cardiac catheterization

    Client 2: A client with a urinary tract infection

    Client 3: A client with an abdominal wound infected with MRSA (methicillin-resistant *Staphylococcus aureus*)

    Client 4: A client with pneumococcal pneumonia

CHAPTER 27 Health Assessment

1. During the general survey, the nurse makes observations and collects data regarding
   - ✓ a. height, weight, and posture.
   - b. blood pressure and urine specific gravity.
   - c. personal hygiene, facial expressions, and lipid profile.
   - d. nail biting, sweating, and complete blood count.

2. Match the term in the left column with its definition from the right column.

✓ __c__	hemodynamic regulation	a. The phase in which the ventricles contract to eject blood
✓ __a__	systole	b. The measurement of pressure pulsations exerted against the blood vessel walls during systole and diastole
✓ __f__	diastole	c. The maintenance of an appropriate environment in tissue fluids
__d__	stroke volume	d. The measurement of blood that enters the aorta with each ventricular contraction
✓ __e__	cardiac output	e. The volume of blood pumped in one minute
__g__	pulse pressure	f. The phase in which ventricles are relaxed and no blood is being ejected
__b__	blood pressure	g. The measurement of the ratio of stroke volume to compliance of the arterial system

3. You assess the pulse of a 1-year-old infant. The normal range of pulse for this infant is
   - a. 60–80 bpm.
   - b. 80–110 bpm.
   - c. 80–170 bpm.
   - d. 100–200 bpm.

4. List three things that a client, who needs to monitor daily weight at home, should be instructed to do.

a. _Same time each day_

b. _Before B/fast._

c. _Similar weight clothes_

   keep a log/journal

5. Which position should a client assume when a rectal temperature is taken?

   a. Supine

   b. Dorsal recumbent

   c. Sims'

   d. Lithotomy

6. Identify the pulse points in the figure.

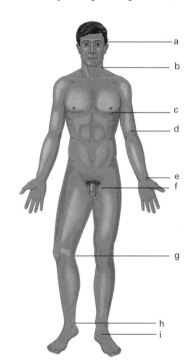

a. _Temporal_

b. _Carotid_

c. _Apical_

d. _Brachial_

e. _radial_

f. _Femoral_

g. _Popliteal_

h. _Posterior tibial_

i. _Dorsalis pedis_

7. Which of the following techniques is appropriate to use when measuring an adult temperature using a tympanic thermometer? Before inserting the probe,

   a. pull the pinna upward and back.

   b. pull the pinna down and back.

   c. pull the pinna down and forward.

   d. pull the pinna upward and forward.

8. According to the Pulse Point Volume Scale, a normal pulse is documented as

   a. +1.

   b. +2.

   c. +3.

   d. +4.

9. Which method of heat loss will result in lowering body temperature when one bathes a child in tepid water?

   a. Radiation

   b. Conduction

   c. Convection

   e. Evaporation

10. Which of the following methods is the proper technique to determine if a client is experiencing a pulse deficit?

    a. Simultaneously have one person count the apical pulse and another person count the radial pulse.

    b. Measure the apical pulse, wait 20 to 30 minutes, and remeasure the apical pulse rate.

    c. Measure the radial pulse in each arm and subtract the difference.

    d. Measure the distal pulse with a pulse oximeter and compare this to the apical heart rate.

11. The term used to describe a respiratory rate equal to or less than 10 breaths a minute is

    a. bradypnea

    b. eupena.

    c. tachypnea.

    d. hyperventilation.

12. Pulse oximetry measures

    a. respiratory effort.

    b. the amount of oxygen in the air.

    c. hemoglobin.

    d. oxygenation saturation.

13. Accurate measurement of blood pressure involves

   a. selecting a cuff large enough to encircle the arm twice.

   b. centering the blood pressure cuff over the cephalic artery.

   c. always inflating the cuff until the manometer registers 200mm Hg.

   d. waiting 2 minutes before taking a second blood pressure reading.

14. During skin assessment, the nurse notices the presence of jaundice. Where does this initially appear?

   a. Nipples

   b. Sclera

   c. Palmar creases

   d. Soles of feet

15. As you review a client's record, you read the notation "PERRLA." Which of the following organs does this notation pertain to?

   a. Eyes

   b. Ears

   c. Mouth

   d. Lungs

16. What does the mnemonic ABCDE mean in the assessment of skin lesions?

   A Asymmetry

   B Border

   C Color

   D diameter

   E elevation

17. The protrusion or bulging of the eye that results from an increased pressure in the eye's orbit is called

   a. paronychia.

   b. nystagmus.

   c. glaucoma.

   d. exophthalmos.

18. Continuous, low-pitched musical sounds heard predominately on expiration over the trachea and bronchi are called

    a. crackles

    b. rhonchi *ir bronspesson*

    c. wheezes *expiration*

    d. stridor

19. In report you hear that your client has hypoactive bowel sounds. Which of the following is the appropriate length of time you would listen to accurately assess bowel sounds?

    a. 15 seconds in each quadrant

    b. 30 seconds in each quadrant

    c. 45 seconds in each quadrant

    d. 1 minute in each quadrant

20. Identify the following cardiac landmarks.

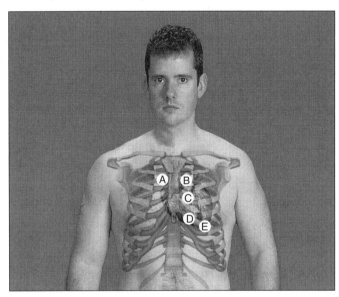

    a. _Aorta_

    b. _Pulmonary_

    c. _Erbs_

    d. _Tricuspid_

    e. _Apical/mitral_

21. The blowing sound that is produced by turbulent blood as it rushes past an obstruction is a

    a. bruit.

    b. thrill.

    c. murmur.

    d. heave.

22. How many kilograms does a 165-pound man weigh?

    a. 363kg

    b. 7.5kg

    c. 36.3kg

    d. 75kg

Critical Thinking

23. During axillary node palpation, a nurse detects a pea-sized lump. Which qualities relating to the node should the nurse document?

    Size, tender/non tender, mobility (more)
    shape, consistency.

CHAPTER 28 Client Education

1. Which of the following statements indicates that a client is ready to learn about diabetes? The client states,

   a. "I will go to the diabetes class tomorrow."

   b. "Tell my wife about my diabetes. She is better at remembering that sort of stuff."

   c. "My doctor tells me I should learn more about the foods I should or should not eat."

   d. "Show me how to inject myself with insulin."

2. Mr. Graves has received his learning materials about caring for himself at home after his surgery. Which of the following methods would best determine that he understands how to care for his incision?

   a. You ask him if he has read the booklet.

   b. You ask him to explain how to care for his incision.

   c. You show him how to cleanse the incision and apply a dressing.

   d. You ask his wife if Mr. Graves understands how to care for his incision.

3. The principles of learning theory state that feedback is most effective when it is

   a. positive and immediate.

   b. negative and immediate.

   c. positive and delayed.

   d. negative and delayed.

4. A client learns how to self-catheterize. Which of the following domains of learning does this represent?

   a. Cognitive

   b. Affective

   c. Psychomotor

5. Organizing content from the simple to the complex makes the learning process proceed in a user-friendly direction. Which of the following learning theorists would subscribe to this principle?

    a. Ivan Pavlov

    b. John Dewey

    c. Jerome Bruner

    d. Robert Gagne

6. When a client is able and willing to learn, the principle of _____ is evident.

7. Match the age group in the left column with the appropriate teaching strategy for that age group from the right column.

_____ children	a. Play imitation
_____ adolescents	b. Teaching the client during the time of day in which the client is better able to concentrate
_____ middle-aged adults	c. Identifying and building on positive qualities
_____ older adults	d. Print-based material at an appropriate reading skill level

8. Ms. Norcross has been diagnosed with hypertension. During her office visit the physician refers her to you for diet and medication counseling. Which of the following phases of care does this activity reflect?

    a. Primary

    b. Secondary

    c. Tertiary

9. A nurse considers the who, what, when, and where of patient teaching in which of the following phases of the teaching-learning process?

    a. Assessment

    b. Identification of learning needs

    c. Planning

    d. Implementation

10. Mr. Canton is being discharged from the hospital in two days. He was admitted for a hypertensive crisis episode due to noncompliance with his prescribed medication regime. Which of the following assessments is a priority in order to determine his discharge planning needs?

    a. His ability to purchase his medications

    b. The cleanliness of his home

    c. The availability of someone to help with his care

    d. The availability of a hypertension education group in his immediate area

11. Ms. Chalahan was admitted this morning with a diagnosis of generalized anxiety disorder. Ms. Chalahan established the following discharge goal with her therapy team: "I will develop and use coping skills to manage my anxiety." Which of the following statements will determine that Ms. Chalahan has met her goal?

    a. "I can cope with my stressors."

    b. "My anxiety level is manageable at a level of 2 on a scale of 1 to 5."

    c. "I know what stress management techniques I need to learn in order to cope."

    d. "My nurse will tell me when I need to calm down."

12. Which principle of documentation pertains to client education?

    a. Documentation may be delegated to a nursing assistant.

    b. Documentation includes only the plan of action and who was instructed.

    c. If the nurse fails to document a teaching-learning event, in the eyes of the law the event never occurred.

    d. Documentation does not require concrete evidence that the desired outcome was achieved.

13. Mr. Greyson, admitted for a bleeding ulcer, has a learning outcome on his client teaching protocol that states, "Client will verbalize signs and symptoms of GI bleeding and report to nurse or MD." After the signs and symptoms of GI bleeding have been discussed with Mr. Greyson, which of the following recordings reflect that the standard for documentation has been met for patient teaching?

    a. Mr. Greyson was taught the signs and symptoms of GI bleeding and seemed to understand the information.

    b. Mr. Greyson was read the materials that described the signs and symptoms of GI bleeding. He said he would take the information home with him.

    c. Mr. Greyson asked about the signs and symptoms of GI bleeding, questions were answered, and he seemed satisfied with the information.

    d. Mr. Greyson was given written information about the signs and symptoms of GI bleeding. It was reviewed with him. Correct responses were given to follow-up questions.

14. Which of the following learning goals is correctly stated?

    a. Mr. Jones will state the side effects of Digoxin.

    b. By his discharge date Mr. Saunders will be able to select from a list of foods those that contain Vitamin K and state which foods are to be avoided.

    c. At the time of admission for surgery, Ms. Barringer will have read her preoperative instructions.

    d. Within one week Mrs. Hanly will learn how to use her walker.

15. It is important that nurses know the reading and comprehension abilities of their clients before using written materials in the education process. Which of the following ratios depicts the number of functionally illiterate Americans?

    a. 1 in 3

    b. 1 in 4

    c. 1 in 5

    d. 1 in 6

Critical Thinking

16. How can the nurse best provide care to clients with hearing or vision alterations?

CHAPTER 29   Diagnostic Testing

1. State three ways in which laboratory and diagnostic testing aid the health care practitioner.

   a. _____

   b. _____

   c. _____

2. *Test sensitivity* and *specificity* refer to

   a. how prevalent the disease being tested is among the general population.

   b. the organisms that are susceptible to antibiotics.

   c. how accurate the test is in screening those individuals with the disease and without the disease.

   d. the type of laboratory equipment used to analyze the specimen.

3. Which of the following methods is considered most reliable when identifying a client prior to a diagnostic procedure?

   a. Asking the client to state his or her name

   b. Checking the arm or leg band

   c. Asking a family member the client's name

   d. Checking the chart that accompanies the client

4. Two factors that contribute to hemoconcentration of blood samples are

   a. _____.

   b. _____.

5. A client, who is receiving intravenous fluid replacement via a vein in her right forearm, is ordered to have labs drawn. Which technique of blood drawing is appropriate?

   a. Blood may be drawn from any vein on either arm.

   b. Blood can only be drawn from the left arm.

   c. Blood must be drawn from the left radial artery.

   d. Blood may be drawn from a vein below the IV infusion site on the right arm.

6. Which step of performing venipuncture is the correct technique?

   a. Wash hands prior to applying sterile gloves.

   b. Apply the tourniquet 3 to 4 inches above the venipuncture site.

   c. Insert the needle into the vein at a 45-degree angle.

   d. Release the tourniquet after you have withdrawn the needle.

7. A port-a-cath is a type of central venous access that is

   a. placed in the antecubital space.

   b. used for short-term drug or fluid therapy.

   c. made from animal tissue and therefore does not need to be heparinized.

   d. surgically implanted under the skin, below the first or second intercostal space.

8. What is the purpose of routine heparin solution instillation in an unused port of a central-line catheter?

   a. To prevent blood clots from forming in the catheter lumen

   b. To prevent the growth of microorganisms in the tubing

   c. To prevent analytes from forming in the tubing

   d. To prevent clotting in the specimen obtained from the port

9. Choose the statement that indicates that a client understands how to proceed with a 24-hour urine collection.

   a. "I will save all of my urine from the time I get up until bedtime."

   b. "If I have a BM, I can allow it to mix with the urine."

   c. "I will drink a lot of fluid so that I can fill up the container more quickly."

   d. "I flushed what I urinated at 6:00 A.M. and will save all of my urine for the next 24 hours."

10. In the white blood cell differential count, which leukocyte is most numerous?

    a. Segmented neutrophils

    b. Monocytes

    c. Eosinophils

    d. Platelets

11. The lab test that reflects the state of glycemia over the past 8 to 12 weeks is

    a. glucose tolerance test.

    b. random serum glucose measurement.

    c. glycosylated hemoglobin A_1.

    d. 2-hour postprandial glucose measurement.

12. Which of the following is a plasma protein that requires Vitamin K for synthesis?

    a. Prothrombin

    b. Thrombin

    c. Fibrinogen

    d. Platelets

13. The creatine phosphokinase isoenzyme that is present in myocardial muscle cells is

    a. Troponin T.

    b. CPK_1 (BB).

    c. LDH_1.

    d. CPK_2 (MB).

14. An individual's risk of developing cardiovascular disease increases when

    a. the triglyceride level is below 200mg/dL.

    b. the LDL cholesterol level is above 160mg/dL.

    c. the HDH cholesterol level is greater than 50mg/dL.

    d. the total cholesterol is below 200mg/dL.

15. Glucose, which normally doesn't appear in the urine, may be detectable when the blood levels of glucose exceed the renal threshold for glucose. What is this level?

    a. 120mg/dL

    b. 150mg/dL

    c. 180mg/dL

    d. 220mg/dL

16. When a client is to receive blood, a type and crossmatch are performed. What is the purpose of the crossmatch procedure?

    a. To determine the presence or absence of A or B antigens in the client's blood

    b. To determine if the Rh factor is present in the client's blood

    c. To determine the compatibility of the recipient's blood with the donor blood

    d. To determine if the Rh agglutinins are present in the donor blood

17. What is the name of the white, chalky contrast medium that is used for roentgenographic visualization of the GI tract? _____

18. Which client has no contraindications for magnetic resonance imaging?

    a. A 54-year-old male who has frequent headaches

    b. A 72-year-old woman with a replacement stainless steel heart valve

    c. A 23-year-old woman with claustrophobia and an anxiety disorder

    d. A teenage girl with multiple body piercing jewelry

19. Parencentesis is the

    a. aspiration of infectious material from the pleural space.

    b. aspiration of body fluid from the abdominal cavity.

    c. instillation of fluid into the peritoneal space.

    d. measurement of pressure of the ventricles of the brain.

20. Your client's blood work comes back from the lab. Among the results you note that the ESR (sed rate) is moderately elevated. What would this most likely be indicative of?

    a. A concomitant elevation in blood glucose

    b. Increased stomach acidity

    c. The presence of an inflammatory process

    d. A folic acid deficiency

21. Match the study in the left column with the organ or body system it examines in the right column.

_____ angiography a. Peritoneal cavity

_____ lymphangiography b. Heart

_____ cholangiography c. Blood vessels

_____ cystography d. Lymphatic system

_____ intravenous pyelogram e. Urinary system

_____ myelography f. Bladder

_____ electrocardiogram g. Biliary system

_____ arthroscopy h. Spinal cord

_____ laparoscopy i. Joint structures

_____ proctosigmoidoscopy j. Rectum and colon

Critical Thinking

22. An adult client's lab work reveals the following: Na 138meq/L, K 3.0meq/L, CO_2 102meq/L, Mg 1.5meq/L. Which of the following electrolyte(s) are not within physiologic range? What common condition(s) could contribute to this alteration?

CHAPTER 30 Medication Administration

1. Which data are essential for the nurse to know prior to administering a new antibiotic medication to any client?

    a. Responses to oral medications

    b. Blood pressure and pulse

    c. Allergies to medications

    d. Weight

2. Which of the following mandates established the United States Pharmacopeia (USP) and the National Formulary (NF) as the official bodies that establish drug standards in the United States?

    a. The Harrison Narcotic Act

    b. The Food, Drug, and Cosmetic Act

    c. The Pure Food and Drug Act

    d. The Kefauver-Harris Act

3. The physician's order reads *Aspirin one tablet qd in* A.M. In the client's medication drawer you find two tablets; one is labeled *Acetylsalicylic acid 325mg*, and the other is labeled *Ferrous Sulfate 324mg*. When you ask a nurse on your unit what the generic name is for aspirin, she replies it is acetylsalicylic acid. Is this the correct answer?

    ❑ Yes

    ❑ No

4. Match each term in the left column with its definition from the right column.

    _____ peak plasma level   a. Maintenance blood level of a drug

    _____ onset of action   b. When the body begins to respond to a drug

    _____ drug plateau   c. Highest blood concentration level of a drug

    _____ drug half-life   d. The time it takes the body to eliminate half of the blood concentration of a drug

5. As you administer nifedipine 20mg sublingually, which of the following instructions would you give your patient?

   a. Make sure you chew the medication thoroughly before you swallow.

   b. Wait a few minutes before you drink or eat anything.

   c. This medication is absorbed in your stomach; make sure you swallow it whole.

   d. This medication must be dissolved completely and swallowed quickly.

6. The medication order reads *Heparin 5,000U SQ b.i.d.* Where in the body will this medication be given?

   a. The dermis

   b. The muscle

   c. The fatty tissue

   d. The vein

7. The bioavailability of a medication administered IM is greater than that of the same medication administered IV.

   ❏ True

   ❏ False

8. Which data will provide the nurse with the most precise measure needed to calculate the correct medication dosage for a child?

   a. Height

   b. Body surface area

   c. Weight

   d. Age

9. Absorption is the physiologic process by which medications are transferred from the site of entry to the rest of the body. Select the statement that best exemplifies this principle.

   a. Oral medications are absorbed rapidly when taken on an empty stomach.

   b. Parenteral medications are absorbed more rapidly than oral medications.

   c. Inhaled medications have a rapid rate of absorption only in clients who are not compromised.

   d. Absorption of medications is dependent on surface area: The larger the area the more quickly the medication is absorbed.

10. Mrs. Kaplan is ordered dorzolamide hydrochloride 1gtt OU t.i.d. Where and when will you administer this medication?

    a. In the right eye, twice per day

    b. In both eyes, twice per day

    c. In the left eye, three times per day

    d. In both eyes, three times per day

11. The physician's order reads *Tylenol 1 tsp q 4h PRN Temp above 101°F.* The medicine cup is marked in milliliters only. How many mL will you pour?

    a. 2mL

    b. 5mL

    c. 10mL

    d. 15mL

12. A medication order reads *NPH insulin 12U SC.* This is an example of a

    a. single-dose order.

    b. stat order.

    c. standing order.

    d. PRN order.

13. The medication order reads *Inapsine 0.625mg IV push q 4–6h PRN for nausea/vomiting.* Your patient needs a dose. It comes supplied as 2.5mg per mL. How much would you give?

    a. 0.25mL

    b. 0.50mL

    c. 1.0mL

    d. 1.5mL

14. List the five rights of medication administration.

    a. _____

    b. _____

    c. _____

    d. _____

    e. _____

15. What is the primary reason for using the air-lock technique when administering an intramuscular medication?

    a. It is used when administering any amount of medication over 2.5cc.

    b. It prevents the medication from staining the subcutaneous tissue in the injection track.

    c. It is used for any medication that is irritating to the tissue.

    d. It is used to prevent leakage of medication into the IM injection track in the subcutaneous tissue.

16. Your assigned patient is receiving all medications via a PEG tube. The MAR reads *Enteric Coated ASA 1 tablet qd via tube.* What is the best course of action by the nurse?

    a. Crush the tablet, dissolve it, and administer via the PEG tube.

    b. Call the pharmacy to see if a liquid substitution is available.

    c. Contact the physician to clarify the order.

17. Which of the following needle gauges represents the largest needle diameter?

    a. 25 gauge

    b. 20 gauge

    c. 19 gauge

18. The medication administration Kardex reads *Neupogen 300mcg SC qd.* Neupogen is supplied as 300mcg per mL. Which of the following syringes would you select to properly administer this medication?

    a. 1mL tuberculin syringe with a 27-gauge needle

    b. 3mL hypodermic syringe with a 20-gauge needle

    c. 3mL hypodermic syringe with a 25-gauge needle

    d. 0.5mL hypodermic syringe with a 27-gauge needle

19. Identify the common intramuscular injection sites and label them appropriately.

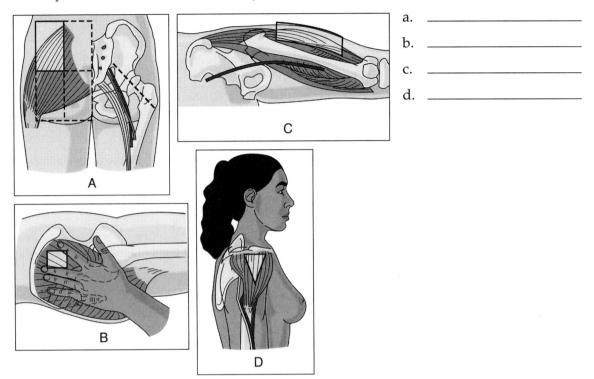

a. _____

b. _____

c. _____

d. _____

20. From which of the following containers would you use a filtered needle to withdraw medication?

    a. Ampule

    b. Multidose vial

    c. Single-dose vial

    d. Prefilled syringe

21. When an IV piggyback medication is administered through a gravity flow system, the primary solution bag is lowered, via extension hook, prior to the start of the medication infusion. What is the rationale for this action?

    a. Ensures that no air will enter the secondary set tubing.

    b. Reduces the risk of microorganisms entering the primary line tubing.

    c. Allows the primary solution to continue infusing during the medication administration.

    d. An increased hydrostatic pressure in the secondary bag causes the primary solution to stop flowing.

22. Which of the following nursing considerations is critical when delivering medications IV push?

    a. The time interval to inject the drug

    b. The port of the IV tubing used to place the medication

    c. The time it takes for the drug to be absorbed

    d. The age of the client

23. While you are assisting your client in using his metered-dose inhaler, he asks, "Why do I have to shake it before I use it?" Which of the following responses would correctly explain this to him?

    a. It makes sure that the two medications are mixed properly.

    b. It activates the medication.

    c. It allows for the medication to mix with the aerosol propellant.

24. The client has a nasogastric tube in place. An oral medication is prescribed. What is the correct procedure for the nurse to follow?

    a. The client should take the medication orally.

    b. Mix the medication with an equal amount of water before administering.

    c. Check the placement of the tube prior to administering.

    d. Flush the tube with 30–60cc of water prior to administering.

25. A mother is concerned that the medication for her 5-year-old only comes in a noncoated tablet form and the child may not be able to swallow it. What advice should the nurse give to the mother?

    a. Crush the tablet and mix in the child's favorite juice or soda.

    b. Place the pill on the back of the child's tongue and quickly close the child's lips.

    c. Crush the tablet and mix it with a small amount of soft food.

    d. Express sympathy and explain to the mother she will just have to make the child take the tablet.

26. A client requires two medications to be given parenterally; the nurse has identified it is appropriate to mix the medications in one syringe. What technique should the nurse use to prepare the medication?

    a. Inject air into vial 1 and withdraw the medication. Change the needle and inject air into vial 2 and withdraw the medication.

    b. Inject air into vial 1, being careful not to touch the needle to the medication. Inject air into vial 2 and withdraw the medication. Change the needle, then insert into vial 1 and withdraw medication.

    c. Inject air into vial 2, withdraw the medication, change the needle, and withdraw the medication from vial 1.

    d. Inject air into vial 1, inject air into vial 2, and withdraw the medication. Insert the needle into vial 1 and withdraw the medication.

27. A client is upset because the pharmacist gave him a generic medication. He is sure it is not the right medication. What is the best way to explain the term *generic*?

    a. It is the name assigned by the manufacturer who first developed the medication.

    b. It is the chemical name given to the medication by the pharmaceutical industry.

    c. It is the name assigned to the medication by the company as its trademark.

    d. It is the name given to medications by the USP and NF.

28. What physiologic principle is important to consider when administering medications to the elderly?

    a. Increased doages may be necessary because the elderly have decreased absorption rates.

    b. Medications are excreted more slowly due to normal physiologic changes in the kidney.

    c. Toxic responses to medications are difficult to measure because of cognitive impairment.

    d. Normal physiologic changes of aging do not necessarily affect dose response.

Critical Thinking

29. The nurse is administering medications to a client. As the nurse is reviewing the medications the client informs the nurse he is not going to take them, because they cannot possibly be the same medications he takes at home. They are different shapes and even the colors are different. How does the nurse respond?

CHAPTER 31 Alternative and Complementary Therapies

1. Ayurvedic medicine embraces the concept of *prana*. *Prana* is best thought of as a

   a. meditative practice.

   b. life force or energy.

   c. transport system for body energy.

2. The field of science that studies the relationship between the cognitive, affective, and physical aspects of humans is called

   a. neuroanatomy.

   b. psychoneuroimmunology.

   c. neurophysiology.

   d. psychobiology.

3. Which of the following groups of physiological responses reflects the benefits of meditation?

   a. Increased oxygen consumption, increased heart rate, and increased blood pressure

   b. Decreased oxygen consumption, decreased heart rate, and decreased blood pressure

   c. Alteration in immune system function, increased levels of lactic acid, and decreased blood pressure

   d. Alteration in immune system function, increased levels of lactic acid, and increased blood pressure

4. Which of the following perspectives on the practice of medicine would emphasize health maintenance and disease prevention through lifestyle choice?

   a. Alternative medicine

   b. Allopathic medicine

   c. Western medicine

5. Which of the following statements best describes the goal of the nurse when the nurse serves as an instrument of healing? The goal is to

   a. provide therapeutic touch to clients when needed.

   b. dispense medicinal herbs useful for a wide variety of ailments.

   c. help the client draw upon inner resources for healing to occur.

   d. help the client access the life force energy in order to facilitate healing.

6. Which of the following complementary/alternative interventions is considered a body-movement intervention?

   a. Tai chi

   b. Imagery

   c. Acupuncture

   d. Aromatherapy

7. Which of the following best describes the physiologic source of the relaxation response?

   a. Increased arousal of the sympathetic system

   b. Increased arousal of the parasympathetic system

   c. Suppression of the parasympathetic system

   d. Suppression of the sympathetic system

8. Sequence the following therapeutic touch (TT) phases in order from the beginning of an intervention to the end of an intervention.

   _____ Evaluation

   _____ Unruffling

   _____ Scanning

   _____ Centering

   _____ Balancing, rebalancing

9. In both therapeutic touch and healing touch, the practitioner uses centering before initiating treatment. Which of the following best describes the process of centering? Centering is

   a. a process of bringing body, mind, and emotions to a quiet, focused state of consciousness.

   b. a process of focusing attention on a client.

   c. a process whereby the emotional involvement between the practitioner and client is genuine and purposeful.

   d. a process whereby the practitioner directs energy toward the client.

10. The massage technique in which the whole hand is used to provide firm, gliding, even-pressured strokes is called

    a. effleurage.

    b. petrissage.

    c. tapotement.

    d. vibration.

11. Which statement best reflects the nurse's understanding of the use of therapeutic massage as a CAM modality?

    a. Massage stimulates the circulatory system; therefore, all patients will benefit from a weekly treatment.

    b. Most clients will receive some benefit from massage as long as they understand the procedure ahead of time.

    c. There are no true therapeutic benefits from massage; it has a placebo effect.

    d. Massage had been demonstrated to be effective for some clients, but is contraindicated for clients with certain problems.

12. An overweight client with a history of noninsulin-dependent diabetes requests a referral to an exercise program. Which intervention by the nurse is most appropriate?

    a. Refer the client to an exercise physiologist or a certified personal trainer.

    b. Instruct the client about nutritional and caloric modifications that will need to be made in response to a change in exercise patterns.

    c. Insist that the client see his physician because nurses cannot recommend exercise programs.

    d. Give the client a list of exercise programs in the community and let him decide which one is best for him.

13. Which of the following is a source of phytoestrogens?

    a. Green tea

    b. Tomatoes

    c. Onions

    d. Soybeans

14. An unstable molecule that alters genetic codes and triggers the development of cancer cells is a(n)

    a. antioxidant.

    b. free radical.

    c. phytochemical.

    d. neuropeptide.

15. Which of the following herbal products, when combined with Coumadin, increases the risk of bleeding?

    a. Licorice root

    b. Danshen

    c. Belladonna

    d. Ginkgo biloba

16. Pet therapy has been demonstrated to be an effective therapy to reduce social isolation and loneliness in which population?

    a. Elderly clients residing in nursing homes

    b. Young children in intensive care units

    c. Middle-aged clients with chronic illness

    d. Postoperative clients

Critical Thinking

17. A 40-year-old client who travels a great deal has been diagnosed with deep vein thrombophlebitis. The client reports receiving weekly therapeutic massages to unwind after a long business trip. What nursing interventions are needed in this situation and what other types of CAM modalities could the nurse recommend for this client?

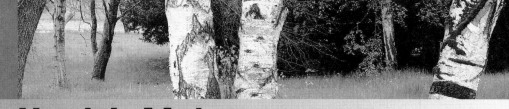

1. Match the term in the left column with its definition from the right column.

   _____ health

   _____ illness

   _____ wellness

   _____ homeostasis

   _____ adaptation

   _____ high-level wellness

   a. A process through which a person seeks to maintain an equilibrium that promotes stability and comfort

   b. The process by which a person adjusts to achieve homeostasis

   c. Functioning to one's maximum health potential

   d. Optimal level of functioning

   e. Equilibrium among psychological, physiological, sociocultural, intellectual, and spiritual needs

   f. Failure of adaptive responses that results in an impairment of functional abilities

2. You note that your client has unmet physiological and psychological needs. Which of the following unmet needs would be addressed as a priority?

   a. Physiological

   b. Psychological

3. Which of the following theoretical perspectives on health would a nurse be operating through when he or she assists a person with the use of health-promoting activities?

   a. Dunn

   b. Pender

   c. Bandura

   d. Rosenstock

4. List three nursing actions that can meet a patient's psychological need for security, a sense of belonging, and self-esteem.

   a. _____

   b. _____

   c. _____

5. A nurse who approaches the client from a holistic viewpoint develops care that focuses on

   a. the individual as a biopsychosocial and spiritual being who is in constant interaction with the environment.

   b. biological manifestations of illness and directs care to remedy the underlying cause.

   c. complex psychological and behavioral integration of health and illness.

   d. the psychosocial aspects and the dynamics of social milieu as part of illness continuum.

6. A nurse who uses Maslow's theory to develop a health promotion plan of care for a client understands that the self-efficacy is closely related to

   a. fulfillment of basic needs.

   b. satisfaction with safety.

   c. self-actualization.

   d. love and belonging.

7. Health promotion programs are best described as interventions

   a. designed to reduce risk behaviors in the population.

   b. that are developed to identify early signs and symptoms of diseases.

   c. designed to assist people to manage daily life stressors.

   d. that assist the individual to achieve optimal health and wellness.

8. A person with an *internal* locus of control feels like a victim.

   ❏ True

   ❏ False

9. Which of the following terms describes an individual's perception of his or her own ability to perform a certain task?

   a. Empowerment

   b. Self-efficacy

   c. Self-concept

   d. Self-esteem

10. Mrs. Evans recently learned that she has been diagnosed with lung cancer. She states, "Why me, why must it be me? I have taken such good care of myself. I don't know how I am going to cope with all of this. Nurse, what should I do?"

    Which of the following responses would best support Mrs. Evans's emotional and spiritual needs?

    a. "I will ask your physician to get a consult with the staff social worker."

    b. "Next time the hospital chaplain is here, I will ask him to stop by to see you."

    c. "Let me get your medications; you will feel better after you take them."

    d. "Tell me more about your situation. I have a few minutes; I can stay and talk awhile."

11. The most effective health promotion strategy a nurse can use to reduce the incidence of obesity in school-age children would be to

    a. direct parents to feed their children a nutritious diet based on principles of the food pyramid.

    b. develop a nutrition education program in collaboration with parents and children.

    c. promote legislation to decrease the numbers of fast food restaurants in poor neighborhoods.

    d. use the food pyramid to teach children how to identify a healthy diet and encourage them to tell their parent what they learned.

12. A nurse makes a diagnosis of ineffective therapeutic regimen management after discovering that the client is unable to purchase antihypertension medication as a result of losing health care insurance. An appropriate nursing action would be to

    a. reassure the client and provide samples of the medications.

    b. assist the client to identify and obtain resources to help purchase medications.

    c. instruct the client about signs and symptoms of hypertension.

    d. notify the physician that the client has decided to exercise and lose weight to control the hypertension.

13. An example of a health promotion activity is a client engaging in a cardiac rehabilitation program after suffering a myocardial infarction (heart attack).

    ❏ True

    ❏ False

14. Disease prevention occurs on a continuum. Which of the following is an example of *tertiary* prevention?

    a. A nurse conducts parenting classes at the local hospital.

    b. The local hospital offers blood pressure screening clinics once a month.

    c. A local health maintenance organization (HMO) offers stress management classes.

    d. A nurse works in a short-term rehabilitation facility assisting stroke patients to regain functional ability.

15. In order for a nurse to be an effective change agent when assisting clients to adopt a healthier lifestyle, which of the following would a nurse incorporate into the care plan?

    a. A standard, unmodified teaching plan for all clients

    b. The client's individual beliefs and motivations for change

    c. Regular appointments for a check-up

    d. Enroll the client in a wellness program

16. Which of the following is an example of an intervention that empowers the client?

    a. Linking a breastfeeding mother with La Leche League International

    b. Arranging for the spouse of a fully functioning client to manage and administer the client's medication in the home environment

    c. Feeding a client when the client is able to feed self

    d. Planning a bathing and grooming schedule for a functioning client

Critical Thinking

17. A 26-year-old client seen in the health clinic complains of stress and reports that his work is consuming his life. In colloboration with the client, the nurse develops a health promotion plan of care. What would be included in the plan of care and how would it be evaluated?

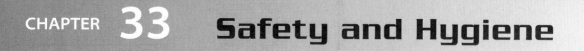

CHAPTER **33** **Safety and Hygiene**

1. A nurse, who is doing a family home care assessment, is told that a 14-year-old boy walks to school on a busy highway. Which of the following pedestrian safety principles should the nurse stress when speaking with the family?

    a. Wear dark-colored clothing to increase visibility.

    b. Use the highway for navigation despite the fact that it doesn't have an adequate shoulder.

    c. Always walk on the right, with one's back to oncoming traffic.

    d. Cross only in crosswalks and wait until traffic has completely stopped.

2. The nurse is preparing to collect a 24-hour urine specimen and requests the lab to send a container to the unit. The collection bottle contains chemicals that preserve the specimen. Where would the nurse find information about the nature of the chemicals that are present in this container?

    a. MSDS: the material safety data sheet

    b. NIOSH fact sheet

    c. OSHA chemical table

    d. JCAHO safety regulation guidelines

3. Exposure to latex may be transmitted by

    a. skin contact only.

    b. inhalation of powder particles from latex gloves.

    c. lipids, which bind to the skin causing dermatitis.

    d. latex gloves, but not other latex-containing products.

4. Using a Hoyer lift to transfer immobile clients is an example of using an engineering control to reduce

    a. technological stressors.

    b. ergonomic stressors.

    c. biochemical stressors.

    d. chemical stressors.

5. When a nurse is caring for a client with an implanted radioactive device, the time spent in direct patient contact is monitored and limited to short periods. This is an example of which type of control measure?

    a. Administrative control

    b. Personal protective control

    c. Engineering control

    d. Nursing control

6. Parents of toddlers are attending a safety education class. Which content, specific to this age group, would the nurse include in the teaching plan?

    a. Toddlers may travel in the front seat of an automobile as long as they have a seat belt on.

    b. Encourage the use of toys such as Legos to improve manual dexterity.

    c. Remove all rugs from the home to prevent falls.

    d. Store all medications in a locked cabinet.

7. Referring to this figure, list the four ways in which clients may become entrapped in beds with raised siderails.

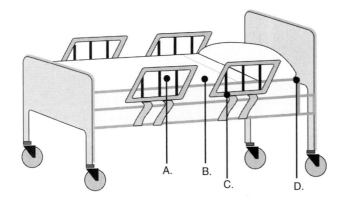

    a. _____

    b. _____

    c. _____

    d. _____

8. Enclosed cloth material applied over the client's hand is a _____ restraint.

    a. mummy

    b. limb

    c. mitten

    d. sock

9. JCAHO restraint standards for nonpsychiatric clients include

   a. monitoring the restrained client every 4 hours.

   b. renewing the order for continuous restraint use every 24 hours.

   c. obtaining clients' written consent prior to restraint application.

   d. using restraints, as the first measure, to reduce client agitation.

10. When a family member of a hospitalized client brings in a TV from home, the nurse notices that the junction between the cord and the plug is loose. The nurse should

    a. wrap the cord with electrical tape.

    b. ask the family to bring in an extension cord.

    c. ask the family to take the TV home.

    d. test the equipment by plugging it in.

11. During a bed bath, the correct procedure used when washing a limb is to

    a. wash the extremity using short, circular motions.

    b. wash the extremity using long strokes in the direction of proximal to distal.

    c. wash the extremity using a back-and-forth scrubbing motion.

    d. wash the extremity in the direction of distal to proximal.

12. While making a bed the nurse chooses to reuse the bedspread because it is not soiled. The nurse should

    a. fan-fold it and place it on the floor.

    b. drape it on the linen hamper while changing the sheets.

    c. fold it neatly and place it on the roommate's bed.

    d. remove and fold the spread, and place it on a clean work area.

13. When handling linen, what technique would minimize the spread of microorganisms?

    a. Rolling soiled linens to the middle of the bed

    b. Placement of seamed side toward mattress

    c. Fanning the linens before placing them on the mattress

    d. Carrying the clean linens against one's uniform

14. Principles of perineal care include

    a. placing the female client in Sim's position.

    b. using a Betadine solution to remove microorganisms.

    c. cleansing the perineum front to back on females.

    d. cleansing the scrotal area with the same cloth used to clean the anal area.

15. When providing oral care for the comatose client the nurse should

    a. turn the client's head to the side, with a basin placed under the mouth.

    b. position the client upright with the head in a centered position.

    c. only administer mouth care if a gag reflex is present.

    d. vigorously brush the client's teeth while wiping secretions away from the mouth.

16. Which action may help to prevent hair damage and painful pulling of the scalp?

    a. Using a firm-bristle, nylon hairbrush

    b. Applying water to the hair before combing

    c. Using a blow-dryer while brushing and styling hair

    d. Massaging the scalp with oil before brushing

17. The nurse is caring for an unconscious client who wears contact lenses. Proper removal includes

    a. positioning the client in reverse Trendelenburg to facilitate removal.

    b. wearing gloves and gently moving the lens toward the cornea for removal.

    c. asking the client to blink while pressing on the temporal area.

    d. flushing the eye with tap water using a 10cc syringe.

Critical Thinking

18. The family members of an elderly client who has been wandering into other clients' rooms, particularly at night, are disturbed that a vest restraint is being used on their parent. What alternatives to restraints could the health care staff try to use with this client?

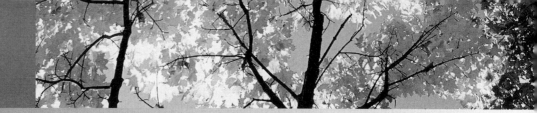

CHAPTER 34

Fluid, Electrolyte, and Acid-Base Balance

1. Match the term in the left column with its definition from the right column.

   _____ solute

   _____ solvent

   _____ electrolyte

   _____ body fluid

   a. The liquid that contains a substance in solution

   b. The substance that dissociates into ions when dissolved

   c. A solution that contains both electrolytes and water

   d. The substance dissolved in a solution

2. Which of the following is the most frequently occurring intracellular cation?

   a. Na^+

   b. K^+

   c. Ca^{++}

   d. Mg^{++}

3. A function of the electrolyte sodium in the body is to

   a. provide strength and durability to the bones and teeth.

   b. regulate vascular osmotic pressure.

   c. regulate the osmolarity of intracellular fluid.

   d. activate enzyme systems within the body.

4. The force that presses outward against a blood vessel wall is

   a. colloid osmotic pressure.

   b. hydrostatic pressure.

   c. osmotic pressure.

   d. the rate of blood flow.

5. Which fact concerning fluid balance and regulation is correct?

    a. Each kilogram of weight lost in fluid represents a loss of 500mL of body water.

    b. The ratio of water to body weight is greater in obese people than in lean people.

    c. In order to adequately remain hydrated while running, one should drink one pint of fluid for every pound lost while exercising.

    d. Insensible loss accounts for 400mL of fluid loss daily.

6. What is the effect of hyponatremia on the brain?

    a. Water enters the cells and interstitial space, causing cerebral edema.

    b. Water moves out of the cells into the extracellular space, causing swelling of tissue.

    c. The movement of water is not affected by low serum sodium.

    d. Aldosterone release by the adrenal cortex is inhibited.

7. Which fact concerning edema is incorrect?

    a. Edema represents the accumulation of fluid in the interstitial space.

    b. Moderate pitting edema is rated as a +3.

    c. The body may retain 5 to 10 pounds of fluid before edema is noticeable.

    d. Peripheral edema may be detected in the lower extremities and sacrum.

8. Red blood cells crenate in

    a. an isotonic solution.

    b. a hypertonic solution.

    c. a hypotonic solution.

    d. a 0.9% saline solution.

9. Ms. Miller is one day post surgery for removal of her thyroid. The nursing care plan indicates Ms. Miller's Chvostek's sign will be assessed each shift. A positive Chvostek's sign indicates

    a. hypocalcemia.

    b. hypercalcemia.

    c. hypokalemia.

    d. hyperphosphatemia.

10. The osmolarity of the IV solution D_5 in 0.45 saline is

    a. hypotonic.

    b. isotonic.

    c. hypertonic.

11. Which of the following assessments most accurately determines a client's fluid status?

    a. Daily weights

    b. 24-hour intake and output calculations

    c. Assessment of vital signs q 8 h

    d. Skin turgor assessment

12. The physician's order reads: "250cc Normal Saline IV, infuse over 3 hours." The drop factor of the macrotubing is 15gtts/mL. How many drops per minute will this gravity flow IV infuse?

    a. 15

    b. 21

    c. 40

    d. 83

13. Your patient has a primary IV infusing of D_5W at 125cc per hour. The physician orders Ampicillin 250mg in 50cc of normal saline IVPB q.i.d. The primary and secondary IV are on a volume control pump. The pharmacy recommends the infusion be delivered in 30 minutes. At what flow rate will you program the secondary (the IVPB) pump?

    a. 50cc per hour

    b. 100cc per hour

    c. 150cc per hour

    d. 200cc per hour

14. An assessment of an IV site of a client who is receiving peripheral intravenous therapy reveals skin that is cool, pale, and swollen. This describes

    a. phlebitis.

    b. thrombus formation.

    c. infiltration.

    d. tissue extravasation.

15. Blood should be infused within 4 hours after initiating the transfusion. Which of the following statements best explains the rationale for the 4-hour limit?

    a. This elevates the hemoglobin and hematocrit levels.

    b. It provides for the client's comfort.

    c. It reduces the risk for the development of hyperkalemia.

    d. It minimizes the risk for the development of a transfusion reaction.

16. Which of the following solutions is appropriate to hang as a secondary bag of fluid to flush tubing that will deliver blood?

    a. Normal saline, 0.9%

    b. Ringer's lactate

    c. 0.45% saline

    d. D_5% in 0.45% saline

17. In order to prevent needle-stick injuries the nurse should

    a. use needleless systems when appropriate.

    b. avoid recapping needles.

    c. dispose of sharps in impermeable containers.

    d. All of these practices will help to reduce needle-stick injuries.

18. The Intravenous Nursing Society recommends that, when flushing an intravenous cannula, the nurse

    a. select any size syringe that is readily available.

    b. use sterile water to flush a peripherally inserted cannula.

    c. use additional pressure when resistance is met.

    d. instill twice the volume of the capacity of the cannula and add on devices for the volume of flush used.

19. Consumption of which food or herb may produce an aldosterone-like effect if taken in excess?

    a. Licorice

    b. Dandelion root

    c. Bananas

    d. Echinacea

20. Identify the parts of the peripheral IV devices.

a. _____

b. _____

c. _____

d. _____

e. _____

Critical Thinking

21. A client who is on intake and output comsumes the following for lunch: 6 ounces of broth, 1 pint of milk, a roll with butter, a fruit salad, and a half cup of Jell-O. Calculate the client's intake.

1. Which of the following is an inorganic nutrient?

    a. Water

    b. Vitamin

    c. Carbohydrate

    d. Protein

2. In a healthy adult, what percentage of total body weight is water?

    a. 20–30%

    b. 40–50%

    c. 50–60%

    d. 60–70%

3. Which of the following nutrients does pancreatic lipase act on in the digestive process?

    a. Carbohydrates

    b. Proteins

    c. Vitamins

    d. Fats

4. Which of the following minerals plays a role in the formation of thyroid hormone?

    a. Iodine

    b. Iron

    c. Copper

    d. Zinc

5. Megadoses of vitamins are recommended in the maintenance of health.

    ❏ True

    ❏ False

6. Match the vitamin in the left column with its function from the right column.

_____ Vitamin A   a. Prevents oxidation of polyunsaturated fatty acids

_____ Vitamin D   b. Promotes the metabolism of carbohydrates

_____ Vitamin E   c. Promotes the oxidation of carbohydrates, fats, and protein

_____ Vitamin K   d. Is a coenzyme to protein and carbohydrate metabolism

_____ Vitamin C   e. Supports retinal pigmentation

_____ Vitamin B1   f. Supports the production of collagen

_____ Vitamin B2   g. Plays a role in blood clotting

_____ Vitamin B6   h. Promotes bone and tooth development

7. During the interview, your client states that she read in the newspaper that antioxidants are good for you. She asks, "Which vitamins can I take that have these antioxidants in them?" Which of the following is the correct response?

   a. Vitamins A, C, and E

   b. Vitamin B complex

   c. Vitamins D and K

8. Excess glucose in the body is stored as glycogen in the

   a. liver and muscles.

   b. liver and pancreas.

   c. muscles and brain.

   d. fatty tissue and muscles.

9. If the body does not have enough carbohydrates, it begins to break down body proteins in order to produce energy. What is the minimum level of carbohydrate ingestion necessary to prevent protein breakdown?

   a. 25–50 grams

   b. 50–100 grams

   c. 100–150 grams

   d. 150–200 grams

10. What is the minimum amount of protein a person must ingest to prevent obligatory protein loss?

   a. 5–10 grams

   b. 10–20 grams

   c. 20–30 grams

   d. 30–40 grams

11. Abdominal girth is a(n) _____ which is used when
    asssessing _____.

12. Assessment data indicate a client has a protein, zinc, and Vitamin C deficiency. For which
    problems is the client at risk?

    a. Impaired wound healing

    b. Cognitive dysfunction

    c. Weakness

    d. Impaired buccal mucosa

13. Using the food groups listed, build the food pyramid from the base up.

    _____ Fats, oils, and sweets

    _____ Fruits and vegetables

    _____ Bread, cereal, rice, and pasta

    _____ Dairy products and meats

14. To assess for Vitamin C deficiency, the nurse would examine the client's

    a. hair.

    b. nail beds.

    c. gums.

    d. skin.

15. The nurse recommends that the client increase whole grains in his diet. Which food would
    be included?

    a. Pancakes

    b. Semolina

    c. Bran muffins

    d. Rice

16. Which of the following assessments would indicate to a nurse that the client's diet could be
    progressed from a clear liquid to a full liquid diet? The client

    a. has hypoactive bowel sounds.

    b. has normal bowel sounds.

    c. reports nausea.

    d. is experiencing severe diarrhea.

17. Which of the following reflects a diet moderately restricted in sodium?

    a. 2,000mg

    b. 1,000mg

    c. 500mg

    d. 250mg

18. Which of the following clients would be a candidate for parenteral nutrition? A client who

    a. can only swallow thickened liquids.

    b. chokes when attempting to swallow foods or liquids.

    c. is experiencing an intestinal obstruction.

    d. consistently ingests 25% of food that is served.

19. Which of the following actions is the proper method to confirm placement of a small-bore feeding tube?

    a. Aspirate gastric contents with a Luer-Lok syringe and check the pH of the contents.

    b. Begin tube feeding which has been tinted with blue food coloring.

    c. Assess breath sounds.

    d. Assess abdominal sounds.

20. The radiologist notifies the nurse that a chest x-ray reveals the client's small-bore feeding tube needs to be advanced 4 inches prior to initiating feeding. On assessment the nurse finds that the guide wire has been removed. Which action should the nurse take first?

    a. Reinsert the guide wire and advance the tube.

    b. Notify the primary care provider the guide wire has been removed.

    c. Alert the nurse in charge so the tube can be advanced.

    d. Tell the client there is a problem with his tube.

21. Your client is ordered to receive intermittent bolus tube feedings q 4h. You aspirate the feeding tube and find that the gastric residual is 200cc. Which of the following actions would you take?

    a. Hold the tube feeding until the residual diminishes.

    b. Place the client in low Fowler's position.

    c. Administer the bolus tube feeding.

    d. Administer the tube feeding continuously via pump.

22. A client is being discharged home with a feeding tube. The nurse teaches a family member to flush the tube with 30cc of water q 4h after feedings and medications. This action is necessary to

    a. maintain adequate hydration.

    b. prevent the tube from kinking after feedings.

    c. clean the tube of residual formula or medication.

    d. make the client feel comfortable.

23. Which of the following actions would be taken before hanging a subsequent bag of TPN?

    a. Draw the serum BUN and creatinine blood sample immediately prior to hanging the bag.

    b. Document the clotting times on the client record prior to hanging the bag.

    c. Mix the lipids with the TPN prior to hanging the bag.

    d. Use new tubing and attach an IV filter prior to hanging the bag.

Critical Thinking

24. A client expresses a desire to lose weight. She tells the nurse she has discovered a new, over-the-counter weight-loss product that will help her lose 10 pounds in 10 days. How does the nurse respond?

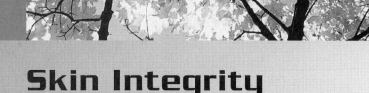

1. The thin layer of connective tissue covering muscle is the

   a. epidermis.

   b. dermis.

   c. fibroblastic layer.

   d. fascia.

2. Nursing actions that can help maintain healthy skin among the elderly include

   a. using alcohol-based cleansing products on the skin.

   b. applying adhesive tape to secure dressings.

   c. using lift sheets for moving and positioning.

   d. applying exfoliating products to dry, itchy skin.

3. Mr. Sullivan is three days out of surgery. During the dressing change you notice that the drainage is thick and yellow and the wound edges, previously approximated, are beginning to separate. Which of the following terms best labels this drainage?

   a. Serous

   b. Purulent

   c. Sanguineous

   d. Serosanguineous

4. A 5-year-old child presents with superficial golden, crusty lesions on his legs and arms. His mother said that he had several insect bites that he kept scratching. What microbe is the most likely cause of this child's skin problem?

   a. *Staphylococcal aureus*

   b. *Candida albicans*

   c. Herpes simplex

   d. *Clostridium difficile*

5. Areas of soft tissue destruction under intact skin that extend in one direction from a primary area of ulceration is called

a. shearing.

b. friction.

c. tunneling.

d. maceration.

6. Skin loss that is confined to epidermal tissue is called a

a. first-degree wound.

b. second-degree wound.

c. third-degree wound.

7. Mr. Church had abdominal surgery four days ago. He puts his call light on and states to the unit secretary, "Something's popped in my belly." Upon inspection you find his wound has eviscerated. Which of the following interventions would you immediately carry out?

a. Call his surgeon and the OR.

b. Apply a dry sterile dressing.

c. Apply a sterile, saline-soaked dressing.

d. Apply pressure using a sterile dressing.

8. During the inflammatory phase of wound healing, capillary permeability increases. This results in

a. decreased blood flow and local warmth.

b. reduction of tissue swelling.

c. white blood cells arriving at the site of inflammation.

d. contraction of the edges of the wound bed.

9. Which client is most at risk for impaired wound healing?

a. A 30-year-old woman with rheumatoid arthritis who takes 15mg of glucocorticoids a day

b. A 40-year-old type 2 diabetes client who maintains good glucose control

c. A 50-year-old male with a surgical abdominal incision who has normal levels of hemoglobin and albumin

d. An 80-year-old male who is malnourished and dehydrated, and whose pulse oximetry reading is 82%

10. Which of the following lab values would you consult to learn what protein reserves are available for wound healing?

    a. Albumin

    b. WBC

    c. RBC

    d. Cholesterol

11. State the four functions of wound dressings.

    a. _____

    b. _____

    c. _____

    d. _____

12. A student nurse who is performing wound irrigation demonstrates correct technique except for one step of the procedure. Which area needs reinforcement by her instructor? The student

    a. wears disposable gloves to remove the old dressing.

    b. holds a bulb syringe 1 inch above the wound for irrigation.

    c. directs the flow of irrigant from the dirtiest area to the cleanest area.

    d. dries the edges of the wound with sterile gauze.

13. A nurse who is removing a client's dressing notices that the gauze is too dry and removal may result in injury to the tissues. What nursing action is appropriate to loosen the portion of the dressing that adheres to the wound?

    a. Pour liberal amounts of saline solution in the wound bed.

    b. Dampen the dressing with sterile water.

    c. Gently pull the dressing and apply sterile gauze to areas of bleeding.

    d. Use a small amount of saline to soften the dressing.

14. Which of the following irrigation solutions would be most appropriate for cleansing a noninfected wound?

    a. Full-strength hydrogen peroxide

    b. Full-strength Provo-iodine

    c. Sterile saline

    d. Half-strength hydrogen peroxide

15. Mr. McGowan is status post coronary artery bypass graft surgery. He has been readmitted to your unit after undergoing a debridement of his infected sternal wound. The surgeon has left the wound open and has ordered wet to dry saline dressing changes q.i.d. Which of the following types of wound healing is this considered?

    a. Primary intention healing

    b. Secondary intention healing

    c. Tertiary intention healing

16. Identify the drainage systems.

    a. _____

    b. _____

17. Which of the following moisture-retentive dressings would you use for a Stage II pressure ulcer which has moderate amounts of drainage?

    a. Transparent adhesive (e.g., Tegaderm)

    b. Hydrogel (e.g., Carrasyn Hydrogel Wound Dressing)

    c. Exudate absorber (e.g., Debrisan)

    d. Hydrocolloid (e.g., DuoDERM)

18. You remove an IV cannula from a patient's infiltrated IV site and direct a nurse's aide to apply a cool compress to this site. You should direct the aide to leave the compress on for what length of time?

    a. 10 minutes

    b. 20 minutes

    c. 40 minutes

    d. 60 minutes

19. Neuropathic ulcers are commonly seen on the

    a. surface of the toes.

    b. plantar surface of the feet.

    c. tibial surface of the leg.

    d. sacral area of the spine.

20. Which of the following assessments is a predictor of skin breakdown?

    a. Stage II pressure ulcer

    b. Persistent erythema of the skin

    c. Blanching when pressure is applied to the skin

    d. Ischemia

Critical Thinking

21. A 15-year-old girl sustained an injury to her knee while playing field hockey at school. Her knee is tender, is swollen to twice its size, and hurts when she attempts to walk. What advice should the school nurse give to the girl and her parent?

1. Match the term in the left column with its definition in the right column.

   _____ incontinence   a. Better rhythmic muscle contraction

   _____ peristalsis   b. Pus in the urine

   _____ defecation   c. Painful or difficult urination

   _____ flatulence   d. Bacteria in the urine

   _____ pyuria   e. Uncontrolled loss of urine or stool

   _____ bacteriuria   f. Evacuation of stool from the rectum

   _____ dysuria   g. Inability to completely empty the bladder during micturition

   _____ retention   h. Discharge of gas from the rectum

2. Which of the following body structures varies significantly between men and women?

   a. Urethra

   b. Ureter

   c. Bladder

   d. Sigmoid colon

3. Which of the following muscles allows adults to postpone urination?

   a. Detrusor

   b. Urogenital diaphragm

   c. Valves of Houston

   d. Depressor

4. Which of the following conditions, if left uncorrected, can lead to urinary retention?

   a. Benign prostatic hypertrophy

   b. Diabetes

   c. Multiple sclerosis

   d. Cystitis

5. Which of the following foods promotes constipation?

    a. Cheese

    b. Chocolate

    c. Celery

    d. Popcorn

6. Mrs. Gibbons, 78 years old, was admitted to the hospital from a skilled nursing facility (SNF) for chest pain to rule out myocardial infarction. She has been in the SNF for two days, increasingly becoming disoriented and anxious. In report you hear that Mrs. Gibbons is unable to hold her urine after she recognizes the urge to void and becomes incontinent on the way to the bathroom. Which of the following types of incontinence is Mrs. Gibbons experiencing?

    a. Functional incontinence

    b. Urge incontinence

    c. Stress incontinence

    d. Total incontinence

7. Clients receiving enteral feedings can experience diarrhea. Which of the following best explains the reason for this?

    a. Digestion is impaired.

    b. The feedings contain a high osmolality.

    c. The feedings damage the GI mucosa.

    d. Clients who require enteral feedings are experiencing a high catabolic state.

8. During the assessment, your client informs you that she takes mineral oil every day to keep her bowels moving regularly. Which of the following nursing actions would you recommend?

    a. Do nothing; mineral oil is a commonly used laxative.

    b. Provide education; mineral oil can interfere with vitamin absorption.

    c. Advise against taking mineral oil; there are less harmful laxatives on the market.

9. The penis of clients who use a condom catheter to manage urinary incontinence must be assessed regularly. What is the reason for this?

    a. To check for lesions or rashes

    b. To check for leakage

    c. To check for twisting of the condom catheter

    d. All of the above

10. Your client is experiencing constipation. Upon digital examination you find the stool is very dry and hard. Which of the following types of enema would be indicated for this patient?

   a. Kayexalate

   b. Oil retention

   c. Carminitive

   d. Antibiotic

11. How would you position a client when preparing to administer an enema?

   a. Left side lying

   b. Right side lying

   c. Prone

   d. Semi-Fowler's

12. Which of the following is most likely to be a temporary bowel diversion?

   a. Double-barrel stoma

   b. End stoma

   c. Ileostomy

   d. Sigmoid colostomy

13. When administering a large-volume enema, the nurse holds the solution set 12 to 18 inches above the rectum for an adult and 3 inches above for a child. The underlying rationale for this behavior is that

   a. at this height, the client is more comfortable because he or she can see the solution flowing by gravity.

   b. this height allows gravity flow of solution without causing damage to the rectal lining.

   c. the urge to defecate is less when the solution is at this height.

   d. administering the solution from this height allows for better cleansing of the bowel.

14. Mr. Stevenson is four days post-op for a colon resection. While you are changing his colostomy bag, you notice the skin barrier has come loose. Upon removal of the skin barrier, you notice that his skin is beginning to ulcerate. Which of the following is the best course of action?

   a. Remeasure the stoma and place a smaller-opening pouch over the stoma.

   b. Cleanse the skin around the stoma with antibacterial solution prior to application of the skin barrier.

   c. Contact the enterostomal therapist for a consultation.

   d. Report these assessment findings to the surgeon.

15. Which of the following is the correct procedure when administering a large enema?

    a. Insert the catheter tip into the anal canal 6 inches.

    b. Instruct the client to hold the enema for 20 minutes.

    c. Ensure the solution temperature is between 99° and 102°F.

    d. Continue the enema administration if the client states cramping is present.

16. During report you learn that Mr. Young has acquired a nosocomial *Clostridium difficile* infection. Which of the following symptoms would you expect to find during your assessment?

    a. Constipation

    b. Diarrhea

    c. Urge urinary incontinence

    d. Hematuria

17. As you interview your client, she informs you that she takes Ditropan for her urge urinary incontinence problem. Which of the following interventions would *not* be included in her therapeutic regimen to manage this condition?

    a. Decreasing the intake of bladder irritants such as caffeine and high acid juices

    b. Adhering to a regular timed voiding schedule

    c. Increasing fluids rich in electrolytes

Critical Thinking

18. The home care nurse is visiting a 76-year-old man who had been hospitalized for a UTI. He was diagnosed with benign prostatic hypertrophy. He now complains of feelings of lightheadedness, especially when he stands. His partner reports the client was given a new medication (Terazosin) by his primary care provider, but they are not sure what it is for and they also want to know if it could be causing the problem. How does the nurse respond?

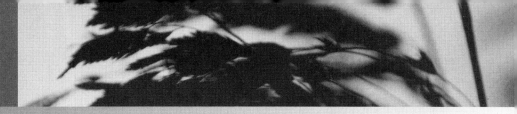

1. The toes are _____ when the foot is placed in dorsiflexion.

    a. pointed downward

    b. spread apart

    c. straightened

    d. pointed upward

2. Which of the following reflects the effects of immobility on the musculoskeletal system?

    a. Risk of thrombi formation

    b. Protein annabolism

    c. Calcium loss

    d. Increased respiratory capacity

3. Increased dietary protein is provided for patients who are immobile. Which of the following statements best explains the reason for this intervention?

    a. This is an attempt at the prevention of pressure ulcers.

    b. Negative nitrogen balance occurs.

    c. Peristalsis decreases; therefore, patients lose their appetites.

    d. There is a tendency for the immobile to form renal calculi.

4. Mrs. Cassidy was admitted earlier this morning with a cerebrovascular accident, with her right side affected. She is confused and she cannot feed herself or wash herself. Based on these assessment data, which of the following nursing diagnoses is the most appropriate for Mrs. Cassidy?

    a. Self-care deficits

    b. Deficient knowledge

    c. Activity intolerance

    d. Risk for aspiration

5. A convex curvature of the spine that is often seen in women with osteoporosis is

   a. scoliosis.

   b. lordosis.

   c. list.

   d. kyphosis.

6. Match each term from the left column with its definition from the right column.

   _____ active ROM   a. Bending of the joint so that articulating bones
                                       are moved farther apart

   _____ passive ROM   b. One body part being across another body part
                                       at least 180 degrees

   _____ active-assistive ROM   c. ROM performed by the client

   _____ adduction   d. ROM performed by the nurse

   _____ supination   e. Turning the body or body part upward

   _____ opposition   f. Moving toward the midline

   _____ extension   g. ROM performed by the client, nurse assists

7. A client who suffered a stroke has left-side weakness. To safely transfer this client from bed
   to wheelchair the nurse will

   a. place the wheelchair on the client's strong side, at a 45-degree angle.

   b. pivot the client on the affected leg.

   c. raise the bed to the highest position to allow the client to slide off easily.

   d. allow the client to dangle for 1 minute to minimize orthostatic hypotension.

8. You hear in report that the head of Mr. Winkler's bed is to be kept in high Fowler's position.
   In which of the following angle elevations would you expect to find the client?

   a. 30 degrees

   b. 45 degrees

   c. 60 degrees

   d. 75 degrees

9. Which of the following types of exercise would you advise a client with a cardiovascular problem to avoid?

    a. Isometric

    b. Aerobic

    c. Isotonic

    d. Isokinetic

10. To safely transfer a client using a hydraulic lift, the nurse must

    a. use the narrowest base of support to maneuver around objects.

    b. center the client on the sling to distribute weight equally.

    c. have client grasp frame of lift for maximum security.

    d. crisscross chains while attaching hook to sling.

11. Identify the two assistive devices being used to aid the client in ambulation.

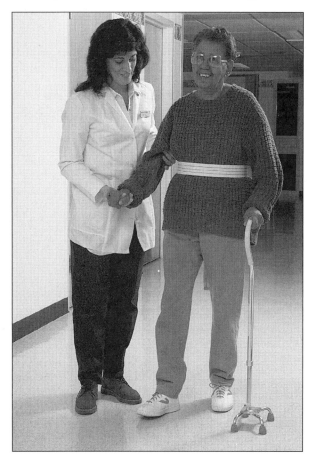

    a. _____

    b. _____

12. A client who requires axillary crutches is being taught how to walk safely with crutches. Which of the following statements is correct and should be included in the teaching plan?

 a. The crutch pad should rest 4 inches below the axillae.

 b. When sitting down in a chair, both crutches should be held on the side of the stronger leg.

 c. When climbing stairs use the stronger leg first.

 d. The elbow joint should be maintained at 180 degrees when walking.

13. Identify the assistive device that the client is using.

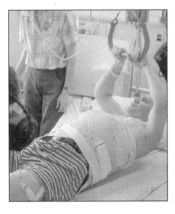 _____

14. While the client is lying in the dorsal recumbent position, feet may develop foot drop. What equipment will the nurse use to prevent this complication?

 a. Trochanter roll

 b. Footboard

 c. Ace wraps

 d. Sequential compression device

15. When lifting an object, bend at the knees, not the waist. What is the principle behind this practice of good body mechanics?

 a. It provides a stable base to lift from.

 b. It is a more comfortable posture.

 c. It provides greater leverage for lifting.

 d. It supports the back muscles.

16. Which of the following crutch gaits is used when one leg is non–weight bearing?

    a. Four-point

    b. Three-point

    c. Two-point

    d. Swing-through

17. Mrs. Duncan was admitted yesterday with degenerative joint disease as a result of her long history of arthritis. Today she had a right total hip replacement (THR). The postanesthesia care unit nurse tells you in report that Mrs. Duncan's hip needs to remain in neutral position. An abductor pillow is in place. What is the purpose of the abductor pillow?

    a. To improve the circulation to the surgical area

    b. To immobilize the hip joint

    c. To ensure that the affected leg does not move laterally

    d. To prevent the right hip from the flexion and extension movement

Critical Thinking

18. The nurse is assisting a client from the lying to a sitting position on the side of the bed. The client states that he feels dizzy and that he wants to place his head between his knees. What action should the nurse take?

CHAPTER 39 Oxygenation

1. Match the oxygenation process in the left column with its function in the right column.

   _____ glottis

   _____ pleura

   _____ medulla

   _____ nasal cavity and nasopharynx

   _____ left lung

   a. Warms, humidifies, and filters inspired air

   b. Has an upper and lower lobe

   c. Closure protects airway from aspiration of foods and solids

   d. Serous membrane covering the lungs

   e. Central respiratory center

2. The oxyhemoglobin dissociation curve is a graphic representation of the relationship between

   a. alveolar and cellular respiration.

   b. aerobic and anaerobic metabolism.

   c. oxygen and carbon dioxide exchange.

   d. the partial pressure of oxygen and oxygenation saturation.

3. A client who experiences a collection of blood in the pleural space is experiencing which of the following conditions?

   a. Pneumothorax

   b. Pleural effusion

   c. Chylothorax

   d. Hemothorax

4. Which of the following medications would be indicated to promote bronchial dilation?

   a. Cromolyn sodium

   b. Albuterol

   c. Beclomethasone

   d. Mucomyst

5. Identify the structures of heart and pulmonary circulation.

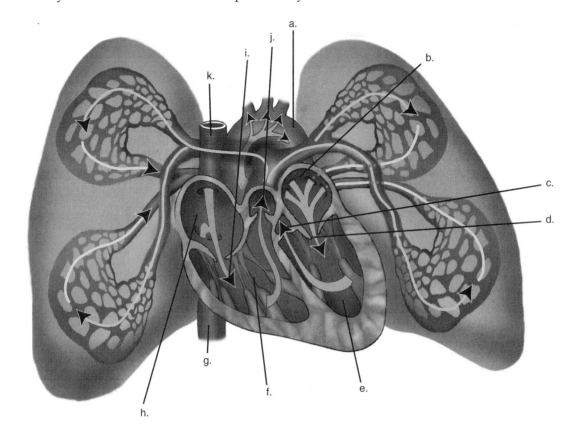

a. _____

b. _____

c. _____

d. _____

e. _____

f. _____

g. _____

h. _____

i. _____

j. _____

k. _____

6. Numerically order the sequence of electrical impulses of the cardiac conduction system.

   _____ Bundle of His

   _____ Sinoatrial node

   _____ Atrioventricular node

   _____ Purkinjie fibers

7. Mrs. Thatcher presents in the emergency room with a chief complaint of pain in her right lower chest and states she is having difficulty "catching her breath." Which of the following open-ended questions would be most useful during the focal interview to elicit additional information about her presenting problem?

   a. How many packs of cigarettes a day do you smoke?

   b. Describe the pain for me.

   c. Tell me what you have had to eat today.

   d. Can you describe your medical history?

8. Which fact related to a child's respiratory system is true?

   a. The epiglottis is short, narrow, and vulnerable to swelling.

   b. Tonsil and adenoid tissue enlarge through adolescence.

   c. The upper airway is shorter and narrower than an adult's.

   d. The number of alveoli at birth is constant through adulthood.

9. What is an acceptable PO_2 level for an elderly adult? _____

10. Cyanosis of the lips appears as a _____ hue among individuals of African American heritage.

    a. blue

    b. maroon

    c. gray

    d. black

11. A common nursing diagnosis for a postoperative patient is *Risk for Ineffective Airway Clearance.* Which of the following interventions would *not* be appropriate for a client with this potential problem?

    a. Restricting fluid intake

    b. Splinting incision during respiratory hygiene measures

    c. Chest physiotherapy every 2 to 4 hours, while awake

    d. Deep breathing and coughing every 1 to 2 hours, while awake

12. A device that an asthmatic client can use to monitor their peak expiratory flow is a

_____.

13. Which of the following is the appropriate amount of suction to use when performing oropharyngeal suctioning?

    a. 80mm Hg

    b. 90mm Hg

    c. 100mm Hg

    d. 110mm Hg

14. Identify the types of artificial airways.

    a. _____

    b. _____

    c. _____

    d. _____

    e. _____

15. Guidelines for tracheal suctioning include

    a. applying continual suction while the catheter is being withdrawn.

    b. suctioning for intervals of 20 to 25 seconds at a time.

    c. suctioning the oropharynx prior to suctioning the lower airways.

    d. providing supplemental oxygen before and after suctioning.

16. When implementing coughing and deep breathing exercises, the nurse teaches the client that its primary purpose is to

    a. change the consistency of sputum.

    b. decrease tidal volume.

    c. prevent hypoventilation.

    d. strengthen abdominal muscles.

17. When teaching safety measures to a client about home oxygen use, the nurse includes the statement:

    a. "Oxygen is a flammable gas and may cause burns."

    b. "Oxygen is not toxic and the flow rate may be adjusted as needed."

    c. "'Oxygen in Use' signs should be posted at entry to home."

    d. "Oxygen is drying to mucous membranes and Vaseline rubbed into nasal skin will relieve this."

18. The procedure for performing the Heimlich maneuver includes

    a. lowering the conscious client to the floor to perform the maneuver.

    b. using a quick upward subdiaphragmatic thrust with an unconscious client.

    c. placing a fist above the xiphoid process and thrusting inward with a conscious adult.

    d. performing a finger sweep on the conscious client to clear the airway.

19. Numerically order the sequence of actions in one-rescuer CPR.

    _____ Open airway using head-tilt/chin-lift method.

    _____ Palpate carotid pulse for 5 to 10 seconds.

    _____ Position client on a hard flat surface.

    _____ Compress chest at rate of 80 to 100 compressions a minute.

    _____ If respirations are absent give two full breaths of 0.5 to 2.0 seconds.

20. The part of an adult tracheostomy tube that is essential for insertion is the

    a. inner cannula.

    b. obturator.

    c. outer cannula.

    d. fenestration.

21. In tracheostomy care, the solution used to clean the inner cannula of mucus debris is

    a. hydrogen peroxide.

    b. Betadine.

    c. one-half strength saline solution.

    d. ethyl alcohol.

22. Identify this low-flow oxygen device.

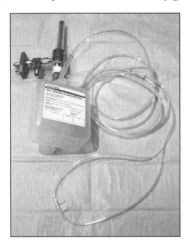 _____

23. This device attaches oxygen tubing to an artificial airway. It is a

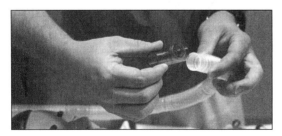 _____.

Critical Thinking

24. A 50-year-old healthy female client who is recovering from laparoscopic surgery has a pulse oximetry reading of 90%. The client is breathing room air and has hemoglobin of 14.3 grams/dL. What is your assessment of this finding?

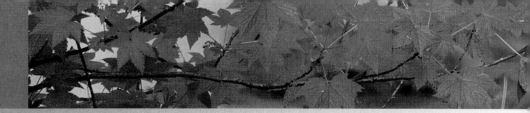

CHAPTER **40** **Sleep and Rest**

1. A client reports feeling stressed and having trouble falling asleep after a difficult day at work. Which action would be most likely to help the client fall asleep?

    a. Go for a brisk walk about an hour before going to bed.

    b. Take dyphenhydramine (Benadryl) about 30 minutes before lying down.

    c. Take a nice warm bath before bedtime.

    d. Enjoy an alcoholic beverage before trying to sleep.

2. The aspect of the sleep cycle which according to EEG is physiologically most like that of the wake cycle is

    a. Stage 1 NREM.

    b. Stage 3 REM.

    c. REM.

    d. Stage 4 NREM.

3. Match the term in the left column with its definition from the right column.

    _____ narcolepsy   a. Manifests by clients sleeping excessively

    _____ hypersomnia   b. Pauses in breathing of 30 to 60 seconds during sleep

    _____ sleep apnea   c. Grinding of teeth during sleep

    _____ sleep deprivation   d. Ssleep walking

    _____ somnambulism   e. Sudden uncontrollable urges to fall asleep during the day

    _____ bruxism   f. Prolonged inadequacy of quality and quantity of sleep

4. The parents of a 5-month-old are concerned that their child takes several naps during the day even though he sleeps through the night. What would be an appropriate response from the nurse?

    a. "Thank you for informing me. I'll report it to the pediatrician."

    b. "You don't need to worry; that is the usual sleeping pattern for an infant."

    c. "You should increase daytime activities that will keep him from sleeping so much."

    d. "Are you sure the infant sleeps through the night?"

5. A 49-year-old client, on the unit for 2 days, demonstrates a change in behavior, marked by grouchiness, general irritability, poor judgment, and a decreased appetite. Her partner reports the client requires 6 to 8 hours of uninterrupted sleep and that has not happened since she was admitted. Which nursing interventions are appropriate?

   a. Request an order for a stronger sedative to help the client sleep.

   b. Plan nursing care to allow the client to have longer periods of interrupted sleep.

   c. Reassure the client that she will catch up on sleep when she is discharged.

   d. Encourage the partner to stay with the client until she falls asleep.

6. A 35-year-old client reports experiencing the inability to move or speak on awakening from a sound sleep. The nurse interprets this condition as

   a. sleep-state misinterpretation.

   b. idiopathic insomnia.

   c. sleep paralysis.

   d. somnambulism.

7. A 22-year-old is being treated for injuries related to an automobile accident. After a few days the client complains of insomnia and reports bizarre dreams when sleeping. Lab results indicate the client was intoxicated on admission. The nurse recognizes the client is most likely experiencing

   a. feelings of guilt following the accident.

   b. REM rebound related to alcohol withdrawal.

   c. NREM disturbance as evidenced by active dreaming.

   d. anxiety about dealing with the insurance company.

8. Parents of a 2-week-old infant report feelings of frustration bordering on anger due to lack of sleep. The nursing assessment reveals they are both getting up when the infant awakens. Which action(s) can the nurse suggest that would be most helpful?

   a. Have the parents take turns getting up with the child so the other parent can sleep.

   b. Instruct the parents to allow the child to cry for longer periods of time before getting up.

   c. Encourage the parents to have a relative stay with them so each of them can get uninterrupted sleep.

   d. Have the parents write down their feelings about the infant.

9. Nursing interventions for the diagnosis *sleep pattern disturbance r/t pain* would focus on

    a. assessing the client's mental status.

    b. pain management.

    c. teaching the client to accept the pain.

    d. developing short-term outcomes.

10. Identify and define two types of involuntary movements that may interfere with sleep.

    a. _____

    b. _____

11. Assessment data reveals that a 45-year-old client snores very loudly. Which sleep pattern disturbance is suspected?

    a. Hypnagogic state

    b. Parasomnia

    c. Hypersomnia

    d. Sleep apnea

12. An elderly client complains about not getting enough sleep at night. Which question will provide the nurse with data that can be used to assess the client's problem?

    a. "Have you been taking a warm bath prior to going to bed?"

    b. "Do you take naps during the daytime?"

    c. "What are you reading after getting into bed?"

    d. "Have you tried exercising before getting into bed?"

13. A nurse has just completed a teaching session for a group of women experiencing sleeplessness related to menopausal symptoms. Which statement indicates an understanding of successful nursing strategies the clients can use?

    a. "It's okay to exercise 30 to 45 minutes before I go to bed."

    b. "Herbal remedies, such as chamomile tea, will help me relax and fall asleep."

    c. "There is really nothing that works. I'll sleep better once menopause is over."

    d. "I should get a prescription for Ambien from my primary care provider; that is the best solution."

Critical Thinking

14. How would the nurse respond to a group of parents who are interested in learning the impact of teenage slumber parties, where children get little sleep, on their child's overall health?

CHAPTER 41 Sensation, Perception, and Cognition

1. Which of the following part of the brain is responsible for maintaining equilibrium?

   a. Cerebrum

   b. Brain stem

   c. Cerebellum

   d. Broca's area

2. Which of the following controls sleep/wakefulness and consciousness?

   a. The glossopharyngeal nerve

   b. The somatic nervous system

   c. The diencephalon

   d. The reticular activating system

3. A client states, "The president of the United States is telling me that I must leave this place." This statement is an example of

   a. an illusion.

   b. a visual hallucination.

   c. an auditory hallucination.

   d. poor judgment.

4. In which of the following situations would the client be at risk for developing sensory overload?

   a. A 10-year-old in the x-ray department waiting for a chest x-ray

   b. A 79-year-old in the intensive care unit recovering from surgery

   c. A 40-year-old, with a chief complaint of a skin rash, being evaluated by a nurse practitioner

   d. An 85-year-old receiving a vitamin injection in her home by a visiting nurse

5. Mrs. Provencano, a 90-year-old resident in your long-term care facility, is hard of hearing, cannot ambulate, and speaks Italian with very few words of English. Her daughter visits rarely because of distance. Her daughter states that her mother feels alone now that most of her friends have died and her family can't visit as much as she desires. Which of the following nursing diagnoses would best apply for Mrs. Provencano?

   a. *Social Isolation*

   b. *Altered Thought Process*

   c. *Sensory-Perceptual Alteration: Hearing*

   d. *Ineffective Family Coping*

6. You assess Mr. Jones's mental status. He can tell you his name but not what day it is or where he is. He knows he has been ill but cannot tell you the reason for his admission. Which of the following nurses' notes would be an accurate documentation of his orientation?

   a. Oriented $\times 1$

   b. Oriented $\times 2$

   c. Oriented $\times 3$

7. As you listen to report on your client, Mr. Lee, you hear that his level of consciousness (LOC) has deteriorated from alert to obtunded. Based on this information, how would you expect to find him when you enter his room?

   a. Nonverbal, unable to follow commands, but does move if stimulated

   b. Unconscious with no meaningful response to stimuli

   c. Slow to respond, drifts off to sleep when not stimulated

   d. Sleeps most of the time, inconsistently follows commands, difficult to arouse

8. Which of the following would you teach a client who is experiencing a tactile deficit?

   a. "Use assistive devices such as a hearing aid."

   b. "Place a calendar and clock in rooms that you frequent."

   c. "Avoid using heating pads."

   d. "Purchase books on tape or books that contain large print."

9. You have placed the nursing diagnosis *Disturbed Thought Process* on Mr. Jubinski's care plan. Which of the following nursing interventions is appropriate to include on his care plan?

   a. Keep the environment calm.

   b. Monitor client closely; check every 30 minutes.

   c. Use physical restraints PRN.

   d. Participate in large-group activities as often as possible.

10. Which of the following nursing diagnoses is a priority for a client who is experiencing an altered level of consciousness?

    a. *Sensory-Perceptual Alteration*

    b. *Risk for Injury*

    c. *Disturbed Thought Process*

    d. *Disturbed Body Image*

11. Which of the following interventions would be appropriate for a client experiencing a visual impairment?

    a. Use brief, concise statements.

    b. Speak in raised tones.

    c. Keep objects in their usual place.

    d. Provide a private room whenever possible.

12. You are assessing Mrs. Tatro. She cannot remember if her daughter was in to visit her yesterday. She *can* remember, with clarity, events from her early adulthood. How would you summarize the quality of her memory?

    a. Recent recall but poor long-term memory

    b. Intact long-term memory but limited recent recall

    c. Intact long-term memory but poor immediate memory

    d. Intact short-term recall, intermediate recall

13. A commonly used nursing intervention is client teaching. Which of the following statements best supports the strategy to delay client teaching when a client's anxiety level is high?

    a. As the anxiety level increases, it interferes with the client's ability to concentrate by decreasing his or her attention span.

    b. During high anxiety periods, efferent nerve pathways are stimulated, which causes a disruption in memory.

    c. Anxiety increases one's ability to perceive certain stimuli; therefore, it does not interfere with one's ability to attend to information.

    d. The ability to concentrate is dependent on a person's prior knowledge, not anxiety level.

14. You read on the client's medical record that the client has "poor impulse control." For which of the following components of cognition does this entry reflect an assessment?

    a. Affect

    b. Judgment

    c. Perception

    d. Memory

15. Which of the following medications would *not* contribute to the alteration in level of consciousness?

    a. Morphine sulfate (analgesic)

    b. Librium (benzodiazepine)

    c. Phenobarbital (sedative)

    d. Insulin (antidiabetic agent)

Critical Thinking

16. A nursing assistant in a long-term care facility asks if it is okay to allow a 76-year-old ambulatory client who, in the assistant's opinion, is only mildly confused to shower independently. The assistant states, "I am so behind in my work. I promise to listen for any problems and I'll be nearby changing the bed linens." What is an appropriate nursing intervention in this situation?

17. A 26-year-old client is admitted to the ER following a motorcycle collision. The nursing assessment indicates the client responds to verbal stimuli by opening his eyes and is disoriented but able to converse. The score on the Glasgow scale is 13. How would this data be interpreted and what are the implications for additional nursing interventions?

CHAPTER 42 Pain

1. The best way for a nurse to determine if a client is in pain is to

   a. observe the client's emotional responses to the environment.

   b. ask the client if he or she is experiencing any discomfort.

   c. ask the medication nurse when the client received the last dose of pain medication.

   d. check the MAR or chart for the last time pain medication was given.

2. Which of the following describes pain originating in the internal organs?

   a. Visceral pain

   b. Somatic pain

   c. Cutaneous pain

   d. Neuralgia

3. The changing of noxious stimuli in sensory nerve endings to energy impulses is referred to as

   a. modulation.

   b. transduction.

   c. transmission.

   d. perception.

4. The four vital signs are blood pressure, temperature, pulse, and respiration. Which of the following is now considered the "fifth" vital sign?

   a. Comfort

   b. Sleep

   c. Hydration status

   d. Pain level

5. For which of the following types of pain would oxygen administration be indicated?

    a. Colic

    b. Ischemic

    c. Neuropathic

    d. Myofascial

6. Which method will be most useful for the nurse assessing the intensity of a 4-year-old's pain?

    a. Asking the child to point to where it hurts the most

    b. Giving the child a chart and have the child point to the number that best describes the pain

    c. Asking the child if his mommy gave him something to help the pain go away

    d. Using the Baker/Wong face scale and having the child point to the picture that best describes the pain

7. Which of the following nursing interventions have a basis in the gate control theory of pain management?

    a. Administering acetaminophen (Tylenol) as ordered

    b. Distracting the client with television

    c. Administering a back massage

    d. Allowing the client to express negative feelings

8. The client who is experiencing pain is also most likely to report which of these symptoms?

    a. Decreased pulse and respirations

    b. Increased feelings of anxiety

    c. Increased blood pressure

    d. High tolerance for activity

9. Mrs. Apperson, age 80, has had arthritis "as long as I can remember." She has difficulty ambulating and says it's because of her stiff, painful joints. She rates her pain most times as a 4 on a 10-point scale. She has gained 10 pounds over the past two months. The staff has noticed that she doesn't ambulate as often as she used to; she says she is afraid of falling. Which of the following NANDA nursing diagnoses would be appropriate for Mrs. Apperson?

   a. Pain

   b. Chronic pain

   c. Acute pain

   d. Fatigue

10. What is the major advantage to the use of a PCA pump in pain management?

   a. The pharmacy prepares the medication.

   b. It is possible to administer more than the usual and customary dose of an analgesic.

   c. The pain management team is responsible for accuracy of the dose prescription.

   d. The patient can control the dosing of the analgesic.

11. Match the pain intervention in the left column with its definition from the right column.

_____ distraction	a.	Application of heat and needles to various points on the body
_____ imagery	b.	Focuses the attention away from the pain
_____ biofeedback	c.	Clients learn to influence their physiologic responses
_____ cryotherapy	d.	Release of blocked energy along certain pressure points on the body
_____ progressive muscle relaxation	e.	Application of minute amounts of electrical stimulation to large-diameter nerve fibers
_____ hypnosis	f.	Cold application
_____ TENS	g.	Leads to a reduction in skeletal muscle tension
_____ acupuncture	h.	A state of heightened awareness and focused concentration
_____ acupressure	i.	Focuses attention on a mental picture

12. Which of the following is an advantage of using the intravenous versus subcutaneous opioid infusion as a route of medication administration?

   a. There is no associated tissue volume restriction.

   b. There is less risk for infection to the insertion site.

   c. It provides more effective pain relief.

   d. It requires pharmacy support in order to deliver the medication.

13. Based on what you know about the "ceiling effect," which of the following statements would you make when educating family members about medicating a child with an analgesic?

   a. If your child's pain is not affected by this medication, it is okay to increase the dose by half.

   b. If your child's pain is not decreased by this medication, stop the medication and call the physician.

   c. If your child's pain is not affected by this medication, do not increase the dose; the effect is the same, but the risk for experiencing side effects increases.

   d. If your child's pain is not decreased by this medication, call the physician for a new medication prescription.

14. Match the term in the left column with its definition from the right column.

   _____ addiction   a. Results in withdrawal symptoms when drug is stopped suddenly

   _____ tolerance   b. Psychological dependence

   _____ physical   c. Client requires a larger dose of medication to achieve the
         dependence   same effect.

15. What can the nurse use to anesthetize a client's skin before inserting an intravenous catheter?

   a. Capsicum topical ointment

   b. EMLA cream

   c. Tiger balm cream

   d. Hydrocortisone topical cream, 0.1%

16. A nursing diagnosis of *Sleep Pattern Disturbance r/t Pain* is developed for a patient following surgery. Based on WHO recommendations for medication use in pain management, what is a priority nursing action?

    a. Get an order to increase the amount of hypnotic medications the client can receive.

    b. Assess the client's response to current pain management regimen.

    c. Increase the amount of narcotic pain relief medication the client is receiving.

    d. Notify the primary care provider that the client is not sleeping.

Critical Thinking

17. A 49-year-old client sustained a comminuted fracture of the fifth metatarsal requiring surgical intervention of a bone graft. The client reports anxiety and fear of post-operative pain. The client reports experiencing severe nausea and itching when taking pain medications in the past. The client is also interested in alternative methods of pain control. What actions should the nurse take?

CHAPTER 43   Self-concept

1. Match the term in the left column with its definition from the right column.

    _____ identity

    _____ body image

    _____ role

    _____ self-esteem

    a. What an individual thinks he or she looks like

    b. Set of expected behaviors determined by family, culture, and society

    c. A person's sense of self-worth

    d. The set of characteristics by which a person is recognized

2. Within which of the following life stages does the self-concept develop and change?

    a. Childhood

    b. Adolescence

    c. Adulthood

    d. All of the above

3. An appropriate nursing diagnosis for a patient undergoing a limb amputation related to the client's sense of self would be

    a. *Risk for Experiencing Self-concept Disturbance.*

    b. *Self-concept Disturbance.*

    c. *Alteration in Self-esteem, Low.*

    d. *Risk for Nonhealing Due to Anxiety.*

4. A nurse has school, family, and work demands and is having difficulty prioritizing which tasks to do first. Which of the following types of role conflict does this situation describe?

    a. Interrole conflict

    b. Interpersonal role conflict

    c. Role overload

    d. Person-role conflict

5. A nurse asks a client the following question during an interview: "What are your strengths and weaknesses?" Which of the following aspects of the self-concept does this question assess?

   a. Body image

   b. Identity

   c. Role

   d. Self-esteem

6. Which statement best describes the relationship between self-concept and stress?

   a. Self-concept determines how the individual responds to stress and stress has an impact on self-concept.

   b. Stressors may affect self-concept, but self-concept does not affect one's ability to handle stress.

   c. The research is not clear about the relationship between the self-concept and stress.

   d. While self-concept may help one deal with stress, stress does not necessarily have an impact on self-concept.

7. Mr. Howard, a 59-year-old patient, was admitted to the unit for a lower GI bleed two days ago. He experienced incontinence of bloody stool on his first day of hospitalization. His PMH is unremarkable; this is his first hospital admission since a car accident when he was 20 years old. He is restless and becomes belligerent with the nursing staff when he is interrupted while on the telephone conducting office business. As you give him his medication he says, "I don't need these medicines; there is nothing wrong with me." Which of the following nursing diagnoses would be appropriate for Mr. Howard?

   a. *Alteration in Defense Mechanisms*

   b. *Self-concept Disturbance*

   c. *Hopelessness*

   d. *Social Isolation*

8. A 16-year-old female has been admitted for anorexia. When you collect the supper tray you notice that she has not eaten anything. When you speak to her about this, she says, "I can't eat; I am too fat already." Which of the following nursing diagnoses would most likely apply?

   a. *Situational Low Self-esteem*

   b. *Anxiety*

   c. *Body Image Disturbance*

   d. *Self-esteem Disturbance*

9. Which of the following nursing interventions is directed at minimizing stress associated with illness?

   a. Verbally instructing the client's spouse about effects and side effects of medications

   b. Allowing the client decision making about timing of care activities

   c. Directing the client to ask the physician about postoperative care during hospitalization

   d. Asking the client how he or she has coped with past illnesses

10. Which of the following goals would be appropriate for a client experiencing *situational low self-esteem*?

    a. The client will experience self-esteem.

    b. The client will state his positive attributes.

    c. The nurse will support the client's weaknesses.

    d. The nurse will facilitate the client's growth.

11. You notice your colleague: She is well-groomed, her posture is erect, her speech is articulate, she is able to maintain relationships appropriately, she is self directed, and she is able to take care of herself. Would you say that she has high or low self-esteem?

    ❑ High self-esteem

    ❑ Low self-esteem

12. In which of the following life stages would an individual's self-concept be most influenced by feedback from significant others?

    a. Childhood

    b. Adolescence

    c. Adulthood

    d. All of the above

13. Which of the following is true about self-concept? It is

    a. an individual's perception of self.

    b. the perception of others about an individual.

    c. the reflection of an individual's achievements.

    d. derived from the expectations of others for an individual.

14. A client undergoing a painful procedure may perceive a threat related to

   a. psychological integrity.

   b. inability to control the situation.

   c. physical safety.

   d. unmet physiological/biological need.

15. The concept of learned resourcefulness is best described as

   a. an ability to endure the trials of life without experiencing ill health.

   b. a set of skills one develops throughout life that helps one deal with life events.

   c. a core set of values that enable one to live a full and healthy life.

   d. a belief system that builds on prior learning.

Critical Thinking

16. A 30-year-old pregnant client is having difficulty accepting the physical changes she is experiencing as her pregnancy progresses. She tells the nurse she feels fat and ugly. She reports being worried that the baby will not be as beautiful as her friend's baby. How would the nurse interpret these remarks? What interventions are appropriate in this situation?

17. A 49-year-old female client reveals that she is afraid of dealing with symptoms and life-changing events of menopause: "My friends tell me it is awful." How would the nurse respond to this client?

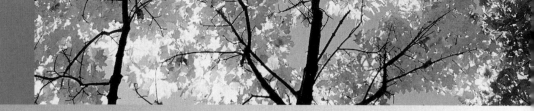

1. Adults who are simultaneously rearing children and caring for elder parents are referred to as the

    a. squeeze generation.

    b. sandwich generation.

    c. in-between generation.

    d. baby-boomer generation.

2. The theory that proposes that families move linearly and predictably through developmental stages in time is the

    a. Family Systems Theory.

    b. Erickson's Theory of Development.

    c. Family Stress Theory.

    d. Family Development Theory.

3. Factors that contribute to social isolation include

    a. church affiliation and being a member of a nuclear family.

    b. being geographically isolated and having brief relationships.

    c. living alone and group membership.

    d. single marital status and constructing long-term friendships.

4. The traits that define collectivism are

    a. relationships that are genetically linked and long lasting.

    b. a member's basic needs being met by the family.

    c. a predominantly agrarian economy.

    d. All of these traits reflect collectivism.

5. Individualism, the predominant cultural type in the United States, predominates

   a. in rural settings.

   b. among cults.

   c. in urban settings.

   d. in developing countries.

6. The family serves two purposes:

   a. _____

   b. _____

7. Research has determined that married couples experience less mortality related to a

   a. motor vehicle accident.

   b. chronic obstructive pulmonary disease.

   c. cardiovascular disease.

   d. depression.

8. Nuclear families

   a. represent 56% of all social units.

   b. evolved as families moved to urban centers.

   c. are associated with an agrarian society.

   d. consist of a married heterosexual couple who do not have children.

9. State three characteristics of a healthy family.

   a. _____

   b. _____

   c. _____

10. A family in which children live with one birth parent and one stepparent is referred to as a

    a. merged family.

    b. nuclear dyad.

    c. Brady family.

    d. blended family.

11. A graphic representation of the family form is called a(n) _____.

12. A dual-career couple living as a nuclear dyad, who share household responsibilities share which of the following family roles?

    a. Provider, housekeeper

    b. Child care provider and housekeeper

    c. Parent, provider

    d. Provider, socializer

13. Match the family function in the left column with the formal role structure in the right column.

    _____ basic need function   a. Provider role

    _____ conjugal function   b. Sexual role

    _____ economic function   c. Kinship role

    _____ health care function   d. Housekeeper role

14. When the expectations of one role are incompatible with those of another role, an individual may experience

    a. role confusion.

    b. role conflict.

    c. role competence.

    d. role overload.

Critical Thinking

15. When a blended family forms, the parent may accept an additional role—the role of parenting stepchildren. What recommendations can a nurse give to a new stepparent in relation to the role of parenting stepchildren?

CHAPTER **45** **Loss and Grief**

1. Match the term in the left column with its definition from the right column.

   _____ actual loss
   _____ perceived loss
   _____ physical loss
   _____ psychological loss
   _____ grief
   _____ mourning
   _____ bereavement

   a. Loss of a body part or body function
   b. Loss of an aspect of self that is not physical; for example, loss of humor
   c. The period of grief following the death of a loved one
   d. An adaptive process related to loss
   e. A series of intense physical and psychological responses that occur following a loss
   f. Loss felt by an individual but not tangible to others
   g. Death of a loved one; theft of an object

2. A nurse teaching a group of teenagers about the concept of loss would use which of the following as an example of situational loss?

   a. A child losing his first tooth
   b. A woman experiencing symptoms of menopause
   c. An executive losing his job due to company reorganization
   d. A teenager moving into young adulthood

3. Mrs. Yankovsky, age 30, is two days post-op for the removal of her uterus and ovaries as a result of uterine and ovarian cancer. The cancer has metastasized to other body areas. Her husband is troubled by his wife's illness; she had previously been healthy. He wanted to have more children. He acts very anxious when the nurses enter the room to give care. Which of the following statements best describes the losses this couple is facing?

   a. Loss of good health, goals, bodily function, and self-concept as a whole
   b. Loss of role relationship, body parts, hope, and job
   c. Loss of a significant other, self-concept, body parts, and support

4. Which of the following theorists stated, "Grief results when an individual experiences a disruption in attachment to a love object"?

    a. Bowlby

    b. Worden

    c. Engle

    d. Lindemann

5. Which of the following phrases best describes a person who has experienced a loss and subsequently does not experience the emotions associated with grief or does not demonstrate the typical behaviors associated with grief?

    a. Uncomplicated grief

    b. Dysfunctional grief

    c. Anticipatory grief

    d. Normal grief

6. Which of the following stages of mourning, according to Engle, would a person who experienced a loss be in for 6 to 12 months? During this time, the person is experiencing feelings of sadness, isolation, and loneliness.

    a. Stage I

    b. Stage II

    c. Stage III

7. Which of the following nursing interventions is appropriate for a 4-year-old child who has recently experienced the death of a parent?

    a. Take the child to the cemetery.

    b. Reassure the child that the child did not contribute to the cause of death.

    c. Tell the child that the fear of death is irrational.

    d. Tell the child the parent is in "a kind of sleep."

8. Mrs. Crowley is hospitalized and dying of bowel cancer. Her husband approaches you angrily, saying that his wife is receiving substandard care. Which of the following responses would be most helpful?

    a. "I understand that you want the best for your wife. Tell me what it is that is bothering you about her care."

    b. "I know it is difficult for both you and your wife, but we are doing the best we can."

    c. "I apologize. We have been understaffed for the past two days."

    d. "I will contact the charge nurse and we will discuss this matter."

9. Matthew, age 6, is dying. He has been suffering with leukemia for three years and is no longer responding to treatment. His mother has difficulty sleeping and eating and feels guilty for not "quitting smoking" while she was pregnant with Matthew. She blames herself for his illness. Which of the following nursing diagnoses is most appropriate for Matthew's mother?

   a. Grieving

   b. Anticipatory grieving

   c. Dysfunctional grieving

   d. Distorted grief

10. Match the Kübler-Ross stage of death and dying in the left column with an example of a client's statement or behavior from the right column that best exemplifies the stage.

   _____ denial   a. The client arranges his own wake and funeral.

   _____ anger   b. The client wants to be left alone.

   _____ bargaining   c. A client states, "Doctor, I want to live long enough to see my daughter get married."

   _____ depression   d. A client diagnosed with heart failure continues to eat foods high in sodium and cholesterol.

   _____ acceptance   e. A client states, "You don't know anything about taking care of someone like me."

11. Which of the following would be most important to know in order to plan for the care of a dying client?

   a. The availability of a support system

   b. The client's oxygenation status

   c. The client's hydration status

   d. The availability of hospice care

12. Which of the following in Maslow's Hierarchy of Needs is a priority when caring for a dying client?

   a. Physiological needs

   b. Self-esteem needs

   c. Self-actualization needs

   d. Love and belonging needs

13. Match the physiological change after death in the left column with the nursing care implication in the right column.

_____ algor mortis

_____ liver mortis

_____ rigor mortis

a. The head should be elevated.

b. Carefully remove tape and dressing materials from the body.

c. Dentures should be inserted, the eyes closed, and the body positioned soon after death.

14. Which of the following is the greatest fear of dying clients?

a. Loss of independence

b. Loss of mobility

c. Pain

d. Dying alone

15. An autopsy would be indicated in which circumstance?

a. A 38-year-old cancer client who dies within 24 hours of being admitted to hospice care

b. A 56-year-old diagnosed with congestive heart failure and complications of type 1 diabetes mellitus

c. A 19-year-old who dies of gunshot wounds to the chest and head

d. A 92-year-old nursing home resident who dies in his sleep

16. An expected short-term goal for a client with a nursing diagnosis of anticipatory grieving would be:

a. Client is able to accept the loss without question.

b. Client verbalizes feelings of grief.

c. Client resumes regular activities within 1 to 2 weeks of loss.

d. Client joins a support group.

Critical Thinking

17. A client is concerned about her elderly husband, whose 13-year-old dog died while he was out of town. The client states, "I know he loved that old dog. He was just like a child to us. My husband is acting irrational; he wants to get rid of his other dog who is 12 years old, and he just sits around the house all day, he won't even go to his favorite coffee shop. He doesn't seem to understand that I am upset, too." What losses are these people experiencing? What signs and symptoms would assist the nurse to determine the stage of grief? What coping strategies can the nurse suggest to assist the client and her spouse?

18. A 51-year-old executive is laid off after 24 years of working for the same company. He is too young to collect retirement benefits and is worried about how he will support his family. He has not been sleeping or eating very well. He has not told his family; instead, he continues to dress for work every day, leaves the house at the usual work time, wanders around town, then returns home in time for dinner. What kind of loss is the client experiencing? What nursing diagnosis and interventions would be appropriate in this situation?

CHAPTER 46

Sexuality

1. Match the term in the left column with its definition from the right column.

   _____ sexuality

   _____ sex roles

   _____ gender identity

   _____ homosexuality

   _____ heterosexuality

   _____ sexual orientation

   _____ bisexuality

   _____ transsexuality

   a. The belief that one is psychologically of the sex opposite to his or her anatomic gender

   b. The human characteristic that refers to all aspects of being male or female, including feelings, attitudes, beliefs, and behaviors

   c. Having an equal or almost equal preference for partners of either gender

   d. How one views oneself as male or female in relationship to others

   e. Culturally determined patterns of behavior associated with being male and female

   f. Sexual activity between two members of the same gender

   g. Sexual activity between a man and a woman

   h. An individual's preference for expressing sexual feelings

2. A client is most likely to provide information about sexual history when the nurse

   a. shares knowledge and information.

   b. is perceived as being open and accepting.

   c. promises not to divulge any information to other health care providers.

   d. acts nonchalantly about the subject.

3. A 28-year-old female client has been diagnosed with breast cancer and will begin chemotherapy soon. She is concerned about her ability to have children. Which response by the nurse is appropriate?

   a. "Don't worry. I have known several women who have become pregnant after receiving chemotherapy."

   b. "Your doctor will talk to you about your chances of getting pregnant."

   c. "I hear that you are concerned. There are several options you can explore such as donating an ova for storage."

   d. "You and your husband can always adopt. There are lots of children who need loving parents."

4. Persons diagnosed with depression may be unable to get pleasure from things that are usually pleasurable. This condition is known as _____.

5. The most important organ(s) for sensual arousal and sexual excitement is the
   a. brain and central nervous system.
   b. breast, especially the nipple tissue.
   c. genitalia.
   d. skin.

6. When instructing teens about sexuality, the nurse should include which of the following information?
   a. Abstinence is the most effective strategy to prevent STIs and decreasing teen pregnancy rate.
   b. Birth control pills are 100% effective in reducing a girl's risk of getting pregnant.
   c. Condoms are the best way to prevent the transmission of all STIs.
   d. Masturbation is a healthy form of sexual expression that helps to decrease STIs and teen pregnancy.

7. A teenage mother reports to the nurse that her 6-month-old infant likes to touch himself when his diaper is off. The nurse informs the mother that
   a. this is normal behavior for a 6-month-old who is beginning to explore his body and developing an awareness of his sexual self.
   b. she should tell the pediatrician about the behavior because the child may have an infection.
   c. it is not healthy for children to play with their genitals because it leads to problems when they get older.
   d. she needs to be sure the infant does not touch anything else and that she washes his hands thoroughly after she diapers him.

8. Medications interfere with sexual function. Those most likely to cause impotence include
   a. antihistamines.
   b. alcohol and depressants.
   c. oral contraceptives.
   d. antihypertensives.

9. When teaching a group of women about prevention of STIs, the nurse recommends the use of a dental dam for which type of sexual contact?

   a. Vaginal-penile intercourse

   b. Oral-penile intercourse

   c. Oral-vulva stimulation

   d. Finger/fist vaginal penetration

10. The nurse has completed an education session related to breast self-examination. Which statement by the participants indicates an understanding of the topic?

    a. "It is best to examine my breasts 2 to 3 days after I have finished my menstrual cycle."

    b. "The best way to examine my breast is in a side lying position."

    c. "As long as I examine my breasts every month it doesn't matter when I do it."

    d. "Using gloves is a good idea; it makes palpating the tissues easier."

11. A client expresses concern that she and her partner will not have a fulfilling sexual relationship after her mastectomy. What information will help the nurse to assist the client?

    a. The age of the client's partner

    b. How comfortable the client and her partner are about communicating their sexual needs and desires

    c. The last time the couple engaged in any sexual activity

    d. Whether the couple have had other sexual partners and how they handled those relationships

12. A mother tells the nurse she is worried that her 17-year-old daughter may be a lesbian because she only likes to be around girls and never seems to date boys. What response by the nurse would be appropriate in this situation?

    a. "Tell me exactly what it is about your daughter's sexuality you are most afraid of."

    b. "Have you told your daughter about your concerns?"

    c. "It is not unusual for adolescents to be interested in members of the same gender. It does not necessarily mean they are lesbian or gay."

    d. "It would be best to discuss your concerns with your husband and then approach your daughter as a team."

Critical Thinking

13. A 53-year-old female reports experiencing pain during intercourse. She reports the pain as 4 on a scale of 10. She describes the feeling as one of dryness and tightness, denies any burning or itching, and has no discharge. She reports that her last menstrual period was over a year ago. She also has not had a gynecological examination for over 2 years. What actions will the nurse take in this situation?

14. A nurse is teaching health educators about issues related to sexuality. In the lecture she refers to the PLISSIT model. Describe the model and how it is used.

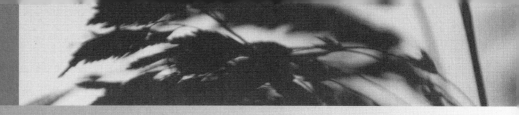

1. Match the term in the left column with its definition from the right column.

__a__ stress	a. The body's reaction to any stimulus
__c__ stressor	b. The ineffective response to stressors
__g__ anxiety	c. Any situation, event, or agent that threatens a person's security
__d__ adaptation	d. The process whereby a person adjusts to stressors
__h__ homeostasis	e. Ineffective coping with stressors
__e__ maladaptation	f. The type of stress that results in positive outcomes
__f__ eustress	g. A subjective response to a threat to a person's well-being
__b__ distress	h. A steady state balancing physiological, psychological, sociocultural, intellectual, and spiritual needs

2. After a particularly stressful day at school, an individual spends a portion of the evening meditating. This type of coping is called

   a. active coping.

   b. restful coping.

   c. delta wave coping.

   d. physiologic coping.

3. The study of the interaction of consciousness, the nervous system, and immunology is called ___Physcho neuroimmunology___

4. Which of the following is a cognitive manifestation of stress?

   a. Impaired judgment

   b. Headache

   c. Insomnia

   d. Social isolation

5. Which of the following signs and symptoms are evident during a fight-or-flight response.

    a. Pupillary constriction

    b. Decreased blood glucose

    c. Decreased cardiac output

    d. Bronchial dilatation

6. Mr. Orapollo, during a routine visit for his diabetes management, states that he is having trouble sleeping, difficulty concentrating, "flies off the handle" at his wife, and cannot find any interest to sufficiently occupy his time since his retirement a month ago. Which of the following type of crisis is Mr. Orapollo most likely in?

    a. Maturational

    b. Situational

    c. Adventitious

    d. Diabetic

7. Which of the following is an appropriate nursing intervention for a client whose anxiety level is severe?

    a. Discuss medication side effects and dosing instructions.

    b. Assist the client in linking the stressor to the anxiety response.

    c. Invite the client to join a group on diet management.

    d. Using broad opening statements, allow the client an opportunity to discuss concerns.

8. The theorist who proposed that the change process occurs in the three stages of unfreezing, moving, and refreezing is

    a. Freud.

    b. Lippitt.

    c. Lewin.

    d. Nelson.

9. Match the defense mechanism in the left column with an example of it from the right column.

f	denial	a.	A nurse comes to work after an argument with her husband and becomes angry with the nurse's aide.
a	displacement	b.	A workaholic mother brings a gift home every day to her child.
e	rationalization	c.	A client blames his wife for misplacing items when he cannot remember where he put things.
g	regression	d.	A student nurse puts his children out of his mind while he is studying for an examination.
d	suppression	e.	A client says he can't follow the prescribed diet because his wife doesn't know how to cook the proper foods.
h	repression	f.	A client with cirrhosis continues to heavily drink alcohol.
c	projection	g.	A 54-year-old patient with bone cancer refuses to feed himself during hospitalization.
b	reaction formation	h.	A client is unaware of her sexual abuse history.

10. Match the system in the left column with its stress-related disorder in the right.

c	endocrine system	a.	Colitis
d	genitourinary system	b.	Eczema
a	gastrointestinal system	c.	Diabetes mellitus
b	integumentary system	d.	Enuresis

11. A single mother of a teenage boy tells the nurse that she can't control her son's behavior and that he won't listen to her about not using drugs. She says, "Well, I guess that's the way kids grow up these days." A nursing diagnosis that is most appropriate is

   a. *Effective Coping.*

   b. *Powerlessness.*

   c. *Denial.*

   d. *Resistance to Change.*

12. Ms. Marrow has come to the emergency room with a fractured right arm. She states she fell down the stairs at home. The hospital records indicate Ms. Marrow has been to the emergency room twice in the past six months for a head concussion and a miscarriage. As you interview Ms. Marrow, you learn she has experienced several losses recently, one of which was the death of her mother. She appears shy and scared. You learn that she is taking antidepressants for "the blues I can't shake." When you ask her how the fall happened, she states, "These things just keep happening to me. I can't stop them." Which of the following nursing diagnoses would be appropriate for Ms. Marrow?

    a. *Ineffective Denial*

    b. *Powerlessness*

    c. *Ineffective Coping*

    d. *Depression*

13. Which of the following phrases explains the benefits of catharsis as a therapeutic intervention for purposes of anxiety management?

    a. Once a feeling is described, it is real and can be dealt with.

    b. It reduces the tension in muscles.

    c. It clarifies the message of the sender for the receiver.

    d. It allows the nurse to offer an opinion on the client's experience.

14. One of the beneficial effects of exercise in managing stress is the stimulation of the production of endorphins. Which of the following best describes endorphins? Endorphins are

    a. a group of naturally occurring, chemically related, long-chain hydroxy fatty acids that stimulate the contractility of smooth muscles.

    b. a group of opiate-like substances produced naturally by the brain that raise the body's pain threshold.

    c. a group of high-molecular-weight kininogens that increase the permeability of capillaries.

    d. intermediate products in the synthesis of norepinephrine, a neurotransmitter.

15. Your client is having difficulty falling asleep. Which of the following stress management strategies would you recommend?

    a. Progressive muscle relaxation

    b. Exercise

    c. Guided imagery

    d. Aromatherapy

16. Match the stress management technique in the left column with its definition from the right column.

    __b__   biofeedback
    __c__   progressive muscle relaxation
    __e__   guided imagery
    __d__   cognitive reframing
    __a__   environmental strategies

a. Noise, sound, light, and other stimuli in the client's immediate surroundings are manipulated.

b. Clients learn to manipulate body responses through mental activity.

c. The client tenses and releases muscle groups throughout the body, paying attention to sensations of tension and relaxation.

d. The client's perception and interpretations are altered by changing of the client's thoughts.

e. A client is guided through a pleasant scene, using all the senses, in order to become fully relaxed.

17. Which of the following assessments would not be useful when evaluating the effectiveness of anxiety reduction strategies?

a. Vital signs measurement

b. Cognition

c. Motor movement

d. Oxygen saturation

18. The nurse admits a visibly anxious client and proceeds to minimize environmental distressors. Which measure would be most effective in decreasing environmental stimulants?

a. Place the client in a ward with four other individuals.

b. Turn on and adjust the radio to a rock station.

c. Allow the client's friends and family unlimited visiting privileges.

d. Personalize the environment with the client's familiar objects.

19. Which of the following hormones is *not* involved in the biological changes associated with the fight-or-flight responses?

a. Adrenalin

b. Thyroid hormone

c. Norepinephrine

d. Glucocorticoids

Critical Thinking

20. A nurse, who has been working on a busy medical-surgical unit for 3 years, begins to have headaches and periods of insomnia. He has been putting in a lot of overtime because the unit has been short staffed. There are times when he works a double shift and returns to work after sleeping a few hours. The nurse is very devoted to his clients and doesn't want their care to be compromised. Which phase of burnout is the nurse experiencing? Which strategies for coping with stress would you recommend to this nurse?

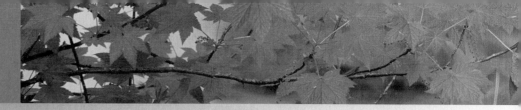

1. The belief that attention to a person's spiritual life would promote healing is attributed to

   a. Clara Barton.

   b. Sr. Callista Roy.

   c. Florence Nightingale.

   d. Dorothea Orem.

2. The mother of a 16-year-old boy, who was admitted to a trauma center following a motor vehicle accident, states to the nurse, "Why did this happen to him? He's only a kid." Which aspect of spirituality is the mother exploring?

   a. Transcendence

   b. Connection

   c. Balance

   d. Purpose

3. The organization that stated a client has a right to care that respects spiritual values is the

   a. American Hospital Association.

   b. Joint Commission for Accreditation of Health Care Organizations.

   c. American Nurses Association.

   d. Patient's Bill of Rights.

4. Among the five variables that typify American religious beliefs, which variable is least embraced by the population surveyed by the Gallup organization?

   a. Belief in god or universal spirit

   b. Importance of religion in people's lives

   c. Membership in a religious organization

   d. Religious preference

   e. Weekly worship attendance

5. Judaism is an example of a

    a. mystic religion.

    b. extremist religion.

    c. prophetic religion.

    d. philosophical religion.

6. The religion that has 1.3 billion members and is the fastest growing sect is

    a. Hinduism.

    b. Islam.

    c. Judaism.

    d. Buddhism.

7. Match the belief or practice in the left column with its religion in the right column.

    _____ reincarnation   a   Sikhism

    _____ the Path to Enlightenment   b. Christianity

    _____ Jesus Christ is God   c. Judaism

    _____ The Old Testament is   d. Buddhism
           the foundation

    _____ The body should remain   e. Hinduism
           intact as given by God

8. Which religion supports the practice of performing "the last rites" for a person who is near death?

    a. Judaism

    b. Roman Catholicism

    c. Buddhism

    d. Islam

9. Blood transfusions are prohibited by which religious group? _____

10. The family member of a client who has just died states, "She will sleep until the second coming of Christ." This belief is consistent with

    a. the Roman Catholic faith.

    b. Unitarian beliefs.

    c. Seventh Day Adventist beliefs.

    d. Quaker beliefs.

11. When a nurse and a client explore the meaning of illness, and the nurse incorporates this insight into the healing process, the client and nurse have formed a

    a. transcultural relationship.

    b. restorative connection.

    c. New Age understanding.

    d. transpersonal caring relationship.

12. The practice of praying for an ill individual by someone who does not have contact with that person is called _____.

13. When an individual's spiritual identity is no longer defined by others, and when one's unique religious identity emerges, this individual is in Fowler's _____ stage of spiritual development.

14. The nursing outcomes classification (NOC) for spiritual distress are

    a. peaceful death, trust, and hope.

    b. dignified dying, hope, and spiritual well-being.

    c. belief in a higher being, faith, and comfort.

    d. tranquility, perseverance, and family support.

Critical Thinking

15. A client who is Roman Catholic asks to be given Communion by a priest who is visiting the unit. The client is receiving intravenous hyperalimentation and is NPO. The nurse understands the importance of receiving this sacrament but is uncertain whether she should allow her client to receive the Communion host. What action should the nurse take?

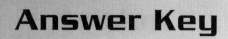

Answer Key

Chapter 1

1. b
2. c
3. b
4. c
5. d
6. a
7. c
8. d, e, c, f, b, h, a, g
9. a
10. d
11. b, d, c, a
12. b
13. c
14. b
15. a
16. a
17. d
18. There are numerous qualities that the early nursing leaders possessed, any of which may influence a student's choice to become a professional nurse.

Chapter 2

1. b
2. b
3. a
4. b, c, a
5. d
6. access, costs, quality
7. c
8. c
9. b
10. aging workforce, fewer persons entering the profession, early retirement
11. b
12. a
13. b
14. c
15. a
16. c
17. d
18. The nurse acts in the role of teacher; provides information about the children's health insurance program, and counsels clients to seek

appropriate prenatal care services through a public health agency. Public health agencies are supported through public funding, and anyone can access the services of the health department.

Chapter 3

1. c, e, b, f, d, a

2. b

3. b

4. developing nursing practice standards

5. b

6. c

7. a

8. b

9. d

10. b

11. a

12. True

13. b

14. c

15. b

16. b

17. a

18. a

19. a

20. Theory in any discipline defines the discipline and what it does. Nursing theory is necessary for the continued development of knowledge and the evolution of the discipline.

Chapter 4

1. a

2. b, a, e, d, c

3. b, c, a

4. d

5. c

6. d

7. b

8. c, a, d, b

9. The nurse is using the visual channel by performing colostomy care on the mannequin, the auditory channel by discussing colostomy care management, and the kinesthetic channel by encouraging the client to touch and handle the medical equipment.

10. Interpersonal communication is occurring when the nurse speaks to the physician on the phone.

11. b

12. c

13. d

14. b, e, d, c, a

15. d

16. a

17. c, d, a, e, b

18. c

19. The nurse can use therapeutic communication techniques to help the client express her feelings and accept the situation. She can acknowledge the client's feelings by using empathetic statements like "I see that you feel sad." She can ask open-ended questions to get the client to open up about her fears and expectations. She can listen actively to what the client is saying. She can sit quietly with the patient and not rush the client.

20. Self-talk is intrapersonal communication of thoughts and feelings that are internal. It is based on one's culture, values, personal experience, and developmental level. Self-talk can interfere with successful communications and can have a negative effect on the nurse-client relationship. The nurse cannot change self-talk, but she can be aware that it exists. The nurse can promote successful communication by approaching clients in a honest, nonjudgmental manner and by accepting the client and validating the client's experience.

Chapter 5

1. a, g, e, f, d, b, c

2. communication

3. a

4. b

5. Respect the client's religious beliefs. Create privacy when the client is engaged in prayer, and appreciate that prayer may influence wellness.

6. c

7. d

8. c

9. d, a, e, c, b

10. Denver Developmental Scale

11. c

12. c

13. d

14. e

15. The nurse may ask the following questions to understand the client's perspective on how SIDS occurs and to develop a culturally appropriate plan of care.

- What is crib death?

- Why do you think placing a baby in a crib may result in crib death?

- Have you or anyone you know had a child who died of crib death?

- Where does your baby sleep?

- What position do you place your baby in when you put the child down?

Chapter 6

1. c

2. d

3. c

4. a

5. b

6. c, a, d, b

7. a

8. b

9. a

Answer Key • 233

10. b

11. c

12. a

13. b, e, d, c, a

14. True

15. c

16. False

17. b

18. d

19. a

20. Nursing research is essential for the development and refinement of nursing knowledge that is used to improve clinical practice. Nursing is a discipline that requires us to know and understand clients and their reactions to their health and illness experiences.

Chapter 7

1. a

2. Computerized infusion pumps, patient controlled analgesia, oxygen saturation, pulse oximeters, pulmonary artery pressure and central venous pressure monitors, ventilators, blood gas analyzers, cardiac and intracranial pressure monitors

3. b

4. d

5. a

6. firewall

7. b

8. Files may be downloaded prior to a home visit; new data may be entered during or immediately after a home visit; the amount of paperwork is reduced and documentation accuracy improved; data may be transmitted to a host computer in a main office or government agency.

9. Holter cardiac monitor, cardiac pacemaker, electrocardiogram

10. CHF, COPD, chronic renal failure

11. In this situation, the health care professional communicates with the client via audio-video monitors. They are able to view and speak to one another and exchange information.

12. c

13. d

14. b, d, e, c, a

15. Bedside computer terminals facilitate more thorough and accurate documentation. Documenting care as it is provided allows the nurse to view trends in physical assessment data that may influence care decisions. Terminals are also used to verify medication orders and access drug information. Quick and easy retrieval of information may prevent medication errors and unfavorable client outcomes.

Chapter 8

1. b

2. c, b, d, a, e

3. 2, 4, 1, 3

4. b

5. c

6. a

7. a

8. a

9. b

10. c

11. a

12. failure to monitor client status, medication errors, falls, use of restraints

13. c

14. b

15. b

16. a

17. b

18. b

19. Encourage the nurse to obtain insurance. The institution may carry a blanket policy, but since the institution may also be sued and will be looking out for its own interests, the nurse will need to hire an attorney who will have the nurse's interest in mind. Also a suit may be filed for an incident that occurred in an institution in which the nurse is no longer employed.

20. The nurse is liable. She is ultimately responsible for the welfare of clients to whom she is assigned. The client sustained multiple injuries. The nurse had a duty to care for the client, and that duty was breached when the nurse did not follow up as planned. The client sustained injury as a result of the breach of duty (cause and effect).

Chapter 9

1. e, a, b, d, c

2. c

3. b

4. b, d, e, f, c, a

5. moral values or religious beliefs

6. informed consent, refusal of treatment, use of scarce resources, impact of cast containment initiatives, incompetent health care providers

7. b

8. d

9. a

10. d

11. b

12. a

13. d, a, b, c

14. a

15. a

16. The nurse has a right to be concerned about the client's HIV status in light of the fact that the nurse punctured his finger with a sharp that was used on the client. However, the nurse cannot coerce that client into giving consent. The Patient's Bill of Rights states that the patient has the right to refuse all treatment to the extent permitted by law, that the health care provider should explain alternatives for care or treatment, and that the patient receive considerate, competent care.

Chapter 10

1. d

2. c, a, d, b

3. b

4. d

5. c

6. c, a, b, e, d

7. subjective, objective, subjective, objective, subjective, objective

8. d

9. c

10. b

11. b

12. c

13. b

14. d

15. d

16. Refer to Table 10-4 on p. 190 of the core book for a thorough review of questions.

Chapter 11

1. d

2. c

3. a

4. a

5. b, a, d, c

6. b

7. d

8. d

9. c

10. 6, 1, 3, 2, 5, 4

11. c

12. a

13. a

14. c

15. d

16. a

17. d

18. Percussion. Used to assess density of structures and to determine location and size of organs.

19. Focal assessment. Ask open-ended questions to elicit information about the client's symptoms: location of pain, character, intensity, timing, and aggravating or alleviating factors.

Chapter 12

1. b

2. for data analysis, as a product or diagnostic label, for an organized classification system or taxonomy of nursing diagnosis

3. a

4. b

5. b

6. e

7. c

8. 4, 6, 3, 7, 1, 2, 5

9. a

10. b

11. It means you should include a descriptive qualifier to make the diagnosis clearer. For example, for "Impaired skin integrity (specify)," if the area of impairment is the left heel then the diagnosis should read, "Impaired skin integrity (left heel)."

12. d

13. d, c, e, b, a

14. a. problem related to
     b. etiology
     c. defining characteristics

15. c

16. c

17. True

18. a

19. The nursing process provides the foundation for the Standards of Nursing Practice in both the United States and Canada. The nursing process forms the basis for the NCLEX licensure exam, and therefore it is essential that the graduate nurse master it. The nursing process provides a systematic method to problem solving and guides the nurse in developing a critical thinking approach to planning client care.

Chapter 13

1. b

2. a

3. d, c, b, a, e

4. 2, 1, 3

5. c

6. b

7. b

8. a

9. b

10. b

11. a

12. b

13. c

14. a

15. a

16. a

17. c

18. Providing adequate oxygenation and relieving his chest pain are the two most critical needs to attend to. They both fall under Maslow's physiologic needs. Once oxygen is administered and an analgesic given, his breathing will improve and pain will lessen. His nausea and heavy sweating, which also come under physiologic needs, should be attended to next. Safety and security is the second tier of Maslow's hierarchy. The nurse should consider that experiencing chest pain and being brought to an ER is a frightening experience. Allaying the client fear should be the next priority. Love and belonging is the third tier of Maslow's hierarchy. The nurse should consider the wife's concern for her husband's welfare and offer her the support she needs. Self-esteem is the next need area to be addressed. The client's desire to take the phone call reflects his need to maintain

self-control. This is a need area that must wait and receives lower priority.

Chapter 14

1. a

2. a

3. d, a, e, c, b

4. d

5. a

6. b

7. b

8. c

9. a

10. b

11. c

12. b

13. b

14. d

15. c

16. d

17. a

18. b

19. The chart is a legal document, and it is the legal responsibility of the nurse to document all interventions and observations to the client's responses to treatments. The nurse cannot delegate that responsibility to the PCA. You can confront the nurse in a gentle manner, ask the nurse to report it to the nurse manager, and explain that you will need to report the incident to the nurse manager. Institutions also use written documentation for billing purposes and for quality control. Written documentation of interventions and evaluation of client responses is an essential communication tool for alerting all health care team members to the client's progress.

Chapter 15

1. b, d, e

2. b

3. d

4. a

5. a

6. process

7. c

8. d

9. d

10. b

11. b

12. a

13. c

14. c

15. a

16. Evaluation of nursing intervention should begin immediately and should be ongoing. Evaluation will ensure that nursing interventions are appropriate and will keep the teaching on target so the client's problems can be resolved

prior to discharge home. Evaluation is also used to determine that learning has occurred.

Chapter 16

1. c

2. b

3. d

4. b

5. c

6. b

7. d

8. d

9. d

10. d, a, f, e, c, b

11. a

12. c

13. b

14. a

15. b

16. c

17. The behavior is inappropriate. The medical record is a legal document. Failure to document appropriately is a primary factor in medical mistakes and is a key issue in malpractice actions brought against health care providers. The chart provides a written documentation of what was done for the client and the client's response to the interventions as well as any revisions to the plan of care. Initially you would talk to the nurse about the

legal implications and the violation of standards of practice. You also need to inform the nurse that you are obligated to report the behavior to the nurse manager on your unit, and then you need to report it.

Chapter 17

1. b

2. d

3. b

4. c

5. c

6. c, d, b, e, a

7. Moro or startle reflex

8. bond

9. d

10. c

11. 6, 7, 2, 3, 1, 5, 4

12. d

13. d

14. d

15. b

16. e

17. The nurse should obtain the child's height and weight and plot the data on a growth chart to determine which growth percentile the child falls in. Once that data is ascertained, knowing that a toddler should quadruple his or her birth weight, the nurse should compare the data with previous height and weight measurements and

evaluate the child's pattern of growth. Assuming that the child is growing normally, the nurse should tell the parent that the child's caloric need is decreasing as his or her rate of growth slows. Many toddlers are fussy eaters and they often eat only two meals a day. Assuring adequate calcium intake is essential for bone growth, and two to three cups of milk will meet this need. Other helpful advice would be to tell the parent not to force feed or use food as a reward. The parent should establish a mealtime routine and allow the child to self-feed. The parent should limit the child's juice intake to 6 oz a day and offer nutritious snacks.

Chapter 18

1. c

2. a

3. c

4. d

5. a

6. hardiness

7. b, c, a, a, b

8. a

9. b

10. b

11. c

12. d

13. a

14. According to Erickson's stages of development, the client is in generativity versus stagnation. The

nurse should reassure the client that his feelings are not unusual given the many changes, including physiological, psychological, and social, that he is experiencing during this life phase. The nurse should encourage the client to provide for his self-care needs, such as developing leisure activities and seeking intellectual activities. Encourage spiritual support and provide counseling for stress management.

Chapter 19

1. d

2. d

3. a

4. a

5. d, a, c, b

6. a

7. a

8. d

9. b

10. c

11. b

12. a

13. b

14. b, c, d, g, f, a, e

15. d

16. a

17. b

18. A decrease in visual acuity, poor vision in dimly lit areas, less foot and toe lift when walking, altered center of gravity, slower reflexes, impaired muscle control, orthostatic hypotension, and urinary infrequency are all factors that may contribute to the high incidence of falls in older clients. The nurse needs to reassure the client that aging does not mean that she is going to fall or need a hip replacement. The nurse should instruct the client in health promotion activities and safety measures that can prevent falls. The nurse should encourage yearly physicals, including eye exams, the use of night lights, and removing scatter rugs in the home. The nurse should encourage the client to take her time when encountering new situations, to use handrails when climbing stairs, and to use assistive devices if necessary when walking.

Chapter 20

1. b

2. a

3. LTAC: long-term acute care

4. CNS clinical nurse specialist, NP nurse practitioner, nurse midwives, and nurse anesthetists

5. connecting with clients, advocating for clients, integrating nursing knowledge

6. d

7. c

8. b

9. d

10. c

11. c

12. Human genome mapping, aging trends, third-party payment systems of insurance

13. d

14. Less than 3 hours must have elapsed between the onset of signs and symptoms and the client's arrival in the emergency room.

15. Evidence-based practice deemphasizes administering a nursing intervention because that is the way in which it was always done, and instead stresses the examination of evidence from clinical research to improve patient outcomes. Nurses will be involved in clinical research at the bedside to determine the most effective means of administering care.

Chapter 21

1. b

2. c

3. a

4. c

5. d

6. a

7. c

8. d

9. The elder has impaired immunity that results in slower healing time and risk for infection. The elder has diminished cardiac and respiratory reserve, resulting in easy fatigability and reduced exercise tolerance. Cognitive processes are slower, and visual acuity and hearing are reduced, which may affect learning new mental and physical skills.

10. b

11. d

12. medicine, nursing, physical therapy, occupational therapy, speech therapy, and social work

13. d, b, c, a

14. c

15. d

16. You should acknowledge the son's concern for his father's health and invite him to attend an interdisciplinary conference, with his father, if his father is in agreement. The son needs information about the nature of subacute care and the services provided. You should tell the son that individuals are assessed as to whether or not they will benefit from rehabilitation, and that the goal, for his father, is to recover as much functional ability as possible.

Chapter 22

1. c

2. state certification, Medicare certification, and JCAHO or CHAP accreditation

3. a

4. c

5. a

6. b

7. Home health nursing care is concerned with restoration and promotion health,. Hospice care nursing is concerned with palliation and comfort when cure is not possible.

8. c

9. a

10. b

11. c

12. b

13. b

14. b

15. Under Medicare guidelines, the nurse's responsibility is to provide care that will ultimately lead to independent functioning of the client and family. The nurse needs to assess the individual's self-care ability and the family's response to the illness. The nurse should include the family and the client in the plan of care, identify external resources that the family and client will be able to use once the client is discharged from home care, and set realistic goals and provide ongoing evaluation of those goals.

Chapter 23

1. b

2. c

3. b

4. c, e, a, b, d

5. b

6. c

7. b

8. occupational health settings, schools, homes, and clinics

9. b

10. b

11. b

12. c

13. b

14. a

15. The community has come to the nurse. Therefore, the nurse has a responsibility to collaborate with the community, using members' expertise to develop a plan that best meets the needs of and uses the resources available to the community. The nurse will be acting in the role of coordinator, facilitator, and counselor in order to assist the community to gain a higher level of health.

Chapter 24

1. b

2. Servant leadership

3. a. Focus is on team members.
   b. Nurses typically work in a team or collaborative environment.

4. b

5. She is behaving more like a manager than a leader.

6. a

7. b

8. d

9. a

10. b

11. d, c, e, a, b

12. b

13. b

14. indirect expenses

15. b

16. communication, empathy, balance, or attitude

17. c

18. A democratic style may be perceived by some as being difficult to follow and understand, especially since staff have been told what and how to do their jobs. It will require staff to develop trust in the leader so they will feel okay about disagreeing without fear of retribution. The decision-making process will take longer because staff will be expected to participate in the process. Ultimately it is the manager's responsibility to communicate this clearly to the staff. Managers who use a democratic style will need to be consistent and fair in their approach to working with staff.

Chapter 25

1. d, b, f, a, e, c

2. c

3. c

4. b

5. c

6. a

7. The nurse's other customers are coworkers and the organization, client's families, visitors, and the community.

8. a

9. d

10. current knowledge base, effective interpersonal skills, caring and compassion, mutual decision making with clients, and individualized care

11. d

12. audit

13. c

14. attending and providing testimony at congressional hearings, writing to ongressional representatives about a particular issue, speaking at civic meetings about particular issues

15. d

16. The nurse manager needs to reassure the new nurse that JCAHO has identified an area of noncompliance and, while it is serious, it is not as severe as a Type I recommendation. The organization has an opportunity to remedy the problem and to submit evidence that it is in compliance with all federal government regulations. The problem must be resolved in a timely manner.

Chapter 26

1. d

2. c

3. b, d, a, c

4. a

5. Objects that have been boiled in water for 15 to 20 minutes at 121°C or 249.8°F are considered clean.

6. Cold water will not cause protein in organic material to coagulate and stick to instruments as does warm or hot water.

7. d

8. d

9. Handwashing; covering of mouth and nose when coughing or sneezing; using medical or surgical asepsis; wearing gloves, masks, gowns and goggles when indicated

10. b and d

11. d

12. b

13. b

14. c

15. d

16. You would give the client with MRSA the highest priority. It is a very contagious organism and may be easily spread through contact. The client with the UTI and pneumonia have no immediate need for a private room.

Chapter 27

1. a

2. c, a, f, d, e, g, b

3. c

4. weigh oneself in the morning before eating, wear similar-weight clothing for each measurement, keep a log of weights, and weigh oneself at the same time each day

5. c

6. a. temporal
   b. carotid
   c. apical
   d. brachial
   e. radial

f. femoral
g. popliteal
h. posterior tibial
i. dorasalis pedis

7. a

8. b

9. b

10. a

11. a

12. d

13. d

14. b

15. a

16. A = asymmetry, B = border, C = color,
    D = diameter, E = elevation

17. d

18. b

19. d

20. a. aortic area
    b. pulmonic area
    c. Erb's point
    d. tricuspid area
    e. mitral area

21. a

22. d

23. Document the size, shape, consistency,
    tenderness, and mobility of the
    palpable node.

Chapter 28

1. d

2. b

3. a

4. c

5. d

6. readiness

7. a, c, d, b

8. b

9. c

10. a

11. b

12. c

13. d

14. b

15. c

16. To accommodate the client's hearing
    loss, the nurse should

    • face the client when speaking.

    • use short sentences and words that
      are easily understood.

    • use signals to reinforce verbal
      information, such as having the
      client handle the medication and
      measure the correct amount.

    • eliminate distracting noises or
      activities from the environment.

    To accommodate the client's visual
    impairment, the nurse should

    • provide large-print material.

- make sure that the client is wearing his or her prescription glasses.

- provide adequate lighting while reducing glare (i.e., do not sit in front of a sunny window while teaching).

Chapter 29

1. Tests can help the health care practitioner evaluate the severity of disease, estimate prognosis, monitor the course of the disease, detect disease recurrence, and select drugs and adjust therapy.

2. c

3. b

4. Prolonged application of a tourniquet during venipuncture, excessive standing time of the sample, and clients with dehydration or burns will all contribute to hemoconcentration of a blood sample.

5. d

6. b

7. d

8. a

9. d

10. a

11. c

12. a

13. d

14. b

15. c

16. c

17. barium

18. a

19. b

20. c

21. c, d, g, f, e, h, b, i, a, j

22. The client's potassium should be between 3. 5 and 5. 0meq/L. The blood work reflects hypokalemia, and one of the most common causes is diuretic use without adequate potassium intake. The other electrolyte values are within normal limits.

Chapter 30

1. c

2. c

3. Yes

4. c, b, a, d

5. b

6. c

7. False

8. b

9. d

10. d

11. b

12. c

13. a

14. right client, right medication, right dose, right route, right time

15. d

16. c

17. c

18. c

19. a. dorsogluteal: gluteus maximus
    b. ventral gluteal: gluteus medius
    c. anterolateral aspect of thigh: vastus lateralis
    d. upper arm: deltoid

20. a

21. d

22. a

23. c

24. c

25. c

26. b

27. a

28. b

29. Tell the client that medications come in many forms—tablets, liquids, and even injectible—and that each company that manufactures a medication has its own trademark style. Reassure him that the medications he is receiving are the correct medications, but that you will double-check the order and the medication administration record to be sure he is receiving the correct medication and dose before administering.

Chapter 31

1. b

2. b

3. b

4. a

5. c

6. a

7. b

8. 5, 3, 2, 1, 4

9. a

10. a

11. d

12. b

13. d

14. b

15. d

16. a

17. Education is key in this situation. The client needs to be instructed that therapeutic massage is contraindicated due to the diagnosis of DVT. The client needs to understand that massage enhances the circularity system and could be detrimental at this time. Other types of CAM modalities that would be beneficial and not detrimental include relaxation, meditation, and guided imagery. All of these modalities have been demonstrated to be effective in reducing stress.

Chapter 32

1. a, f, d, e, b, c

2. a

3. b

4. treat client as a unique individual; protect privacy and confidentiality;

use touch and personal space in a therapeutic manner; respect cultural differences; and decrease anxiety through stress management techniques

5. a

6. c

7. d

8. False

9. b

10. d

11. b

12. b

13. False

14. d

15. b

16. a

17. Initially the nurse must assess the client's overall health status. Then the nurse will identify potential resources and hobbies that the client has access to or likes to do that would enable him to focus less on work. It is important that the client develops diversional activities. Short-term outcome would be for the client to identify two or more diversional activities that he enjoys. A long-term outcome would be that the client actively engage in two activities at least twice a week. Evaluation would be based on client self-report that he is no longer feeling stressed and that he is engaging in the activities as planned.

Chapter 33

1. d

2. a

3. b

4. b

5. a

6. d

7. a. through the bars of an individual siderail
   b. through the space between split siderail
   c. between the siderail and the mattress
   d. between the headboard and the mattress

8. c

9. b

10. c

11. d

12. d

13. a

14. c

15. a

16. b

17. b

18. First the client must be assessed to determine the cause of the wandering. Client safety and the comfort of other clients is of prime consideration. The client should be placed in a room close to the nurses' station and, if the bed has an exit alarm system, it should be

activated. Measures should be used to orient the client to the day-night variations. A night light should be on, the bed placed in the low position, distracting noises eliminated, and toileting needs should be taken care of. The family should be asked what the client's normal bedtime routines are, and the staff should try to maintain them. If a member of the family is willing to stay with the client through the night, the familiarity of a loved one may help to reassure the client and stop the wandering.

Chapter 34

1. d, a, b, c

2. b

3. b

4. b

5. c

6. a

7. b

8. b

9. a

10. c

11. a

12. b

13. b

14. c

15. c

16. a

17. d

18. d

19. a

20.
    a. wings
    b. tubing
    c. stylet
    d. cannula
    e. needle

21. The client consumed 26 ounces of fluid: 6 ounces of broth, 16 ounces of milk, and 4 ounces of Jell-O. One ounce equals 30mL, so the intake is documented as 780mL ($26 \times 30 = 780$).

Chapter 35

1. a

2. d

3. d

4. a

5. False

6. e, h, a, g, f, b, c, d

7. a

8. a

9. b

10. c

11. anthropometric, abdominal distention

12. a

13. 3, 2, 4, 1

14. c

15. c

16. b

17. b

18. c

19. a

20. b

21. a

22. c

23. d

24. The nurse needs to validate the client's proactive desire to lose weight. She needs to educate the client about the fallacy of quick-weight-loss schemes. The nurse begins with a nutritional assessment of the client, then should provide counseling about proper nutrition using the food guide pyramid and healthy eating index.

Chapter 36

1. d

2. c

3. b

4. a

5. c

6. a

7. c

8. c

9. d

10. a

11. a. absorption of wound exudate
    b. maintenance of a moist wound surface
    c. protection of the healing wound from trauma and bacterial invasion
    d. insulation

12. c

13. d

14. c

15. c

16. a. Hemovac
    b. Jackson-Pratt

17. d

18. b

19. b

20. b

21. The injury is most likely a sprain, involving trauma to the supporting structures around the knee. Damage to fibers within the tendons and ligaments often result in swelling, pain, and, in some cases, bleeding. Using the mnemonic RICE (rest, ice, compression, elevation), the nurse should advise the girl to rest the limb by using a crutch for walking, apply ice to reduce the swelling and local bleeding, and take nonsteroidal anti-inflammatory drugs to reduce inflammation and promote comfort. Compression may be achieved by the use of an elastic wrap and the nurse should apply the wrap without compromising circulation. Elevation of the extremity is essential; this will reduce swelling, promote blood flow, and contribute to healing. The symptoms should resolve in 24 to 72 hours. If the symptoms persist or worsen, the girl should be evaluated by a doctor.

Chapter 37

1. e, a, f, h, b, d, c, g

2. a

3. a

4. a

5. a

6. a

7. b

8. b

9. d

10. b

11. a

12. a

13. b

14. c

15. c

16. b

17. c

18. The nurse needs to take a complete history. She needs to complete a physical assessment, including the client's blood pressure lying, sitting, and standing. She needs to assess all medications to determine whether the medications are causing the client to experience the symptoms he describes. It is appropriate to teach the client the use and side effects of the medication Terazosin, which is an alpha-adrenergic blocker used to treat BPH. It works by blocking alpha fibers at the bladder neck and sphincter, causing decreased tone and thereby improving voiding in men with mild obstructive disease. The nurse should also contact the primary care provider since the client will need close monitoring of his B/P and will need titration of his medication.

Chapter 38

1. d

2. c

3. b

4. a

5. d

6. c, d, g, f, e, b, a

7. a

8. d

9. a

10. b

11. a. quad cane
    b. gait belt

12. c

13. overhead trapeze

14. b

15. c

16. b

17. c

18. The nurse should remain with the client and tell him not to move his head forward, as this may cause him to fall. The client should be allowed to dangle his legs over the side of the bed for several minutes, while the nurse places a hand on his shoulder to stabilize him.

The nurse should check his pulse rate and rhythm, and note any changes from baseline. When one is lying down for a period of time, blood pools in the venous system and the autonomic nervous system has to adjust to the position change by signaling the vessels to vasoconstrict. Once the vascular system adjusts, the client will no longer feel faint and can be safely transferred.

Chapter 39

1. c, d, e, a, b

2. d

3. d

4. b

5. a. aorta
   b. left atrium
   c. aortic valve
   d. mitral valve
   e. left ventricle
   f. right ventricle
   g. inferior vena cava
   h. right atrium
   i. tricuspid valve
   j. pulmonic valve
   k. superior vena cava

6. 3, 1, 2, 4

7. b

8. c

9. Any level above 80mm Hg is acceptable.

10. c

11. a

12. peak flow meter

13. a

14. a. oral airway
    b. endotracheal tube
    c. nasal trumpet
    d. tracheostomy tube
    e. pediatric tracheostomy tube

15. d

16. c

17. c

18. b

19. 2, 4, 1, 5, 3

20. b

21. a

22. nasal cannula

23. T-piece

24. Pulse oximeter uses light wavelengths to measure oxyhemoglobin saturation. In a healthy 50-year-old, the normal oxygen saturation should be equal to or greater than 95%. This client is breathing room air, which is equivalent to 21% O_2. She is recovering from surgery, where she may have had general anesthesia. The drugs used in delivering anesthesia may affect oxygenation. The client's hemoglobin is normal, so there are adequate heme molecules to carry oxygen. A reading of 90% typically reflects a PO_2 of around 60mm Hg. This client needs supplemental oxygen, in the form of a low-flow system. A nasal cannula or face mask at 24% to 28% will most likely improve tissue oxygenation and raise the pulse oximetry reading to mid to high nineties.

Chapter 40

1. c

2. c

3. e, a, b, f, d, c

4. b

5. b

6. c

7. b

8. a

9. b

10. a. restless leg syndrome (RLS): creepy-crawly sensations in the legs that interfere with sleep
    b. periodic limb movement syndrome (PLMS): uncontrolled movement of some or all extremities during sleep

11. d

12. b

13. b

14. Teenagers have a high sleep need because of hormonal changes and stress. It is especially important for teens to progress through Stage 3 of the NREM sleep cycle, because this is the period in which growth hormone secretion is at its peak. Growth hormone is necessary for normal growth and also for tissue repair. Encourage parents to have their teens rest before going to an overnight party and ensure the teen gets adequate rest and sleep after the event.

Chapter 41

1. c

2. d

3. c

4. b

5. a

6. a

7. d

8. c

9. a

10. b

11. c

12. b

13. a

14. b

15. d

16. It is not appropriate for a confused patient to be left alone. The patient requires supervision at all times to ensure his or her safety, especially in the shower, where the patient is at risk for falls. It is also important for the nurse to recognize that it is the nurse's responsibility to assess the patient, make appropriate nursing diagnosis, and develop the plan of care. The nurse can delegate tasks to the assistant, but the nurse is ultimately responsible for the care the patient receives. The nurse needs to adequately supervise the assistant and provide guidance and teaching to the assistant regarding how to care for a confused patient.

17. A score of 15 on the Glasgow coma scale, an objective tool used to assess a person's level of consciousness (LOC), would indicate the client is a fully oriented person. However, since there is a two-point deficit in the total score, the nurse needs to continue to assess the client's overall neurological status as well as LOC. The nurse must report any changes in the client's mental status.

Chapter 42

1. b

2. a

3. b

4. d

5. b

6. d

7. c

8. b

9. b

10. d

11. b, i, c, f, g, h, e, a, d

12. a

13. c

14. b, c, a

15. b

16. c

17. The nurse should take a compete history of medications the client has taken for pain relief and the side effects the client has experienced. The nurse can instruct the client about medications that are used in conjunction with the pain medications to alleviate the symptoms the client reports. As a member of the health care team, the nurse can act as advocate for the client, requesting that adjuvant medications such as an antihistamine be prescribed that will help alleviate the symptoms the client experiences. Finally, the nurse can teach the client about alternative methods of pain control, such as relaxation techniques, biofeedback, and hypnosis as well as the use of herbal remedies like chamomile tea, which acts as an anti-inflammatory agent.

Chapter 43

1. d, a, b, c

2. d

3. a

4. c

5. d

6. a

7. b

8. c

9. b

10. b

11. b

12. a

13. a

14. c

15. b

16. Pregnancy is a developmental process that affects all aspects of one's self-concept: identity, body image, self-esteem, and role expectations. The nurse should be aware that the client who is having difficulty dealing with the physical changes of pregnancy may have other self-concept issues that need to be addressed. The nurse can assess the client's expectations of herself and of the baby, and provide anticipatory guidance for the patient as she continues through the pregnancy period regarding additional physical and emotional changes the client may experience, including role changes and revised self concept as she approaches the role of being a mother and parent.

17. The meaning of this developmental transition period is different for each individual; therefore, before responding to the patient, the nurse needs to assess the meaning of menopause for this patient and the patient's knowledge of the menopausal process. Then the nurse can educate and counsel the client about the facts and myths and/or misconceptions of menopause.

Chapter 44

1. b

2. d

3. b

4. d

5. c

6. a. to serve as a social institution to socialize children
   b. to serve the needs of the individual family members

7. c

8. b

9. strong communication skills, time spent together, respect for individuality, trust among family members, adequate play and leisure time, reciprocal social support

10. d

11. genogram

12. a

13. d, b, a, c

14. b

15. The nurse should encourage the new stepparent to be patient with stepchildren and to avoid criticism of the estranged parent. The nurse may advise that the biologic parent and biologic children spend time alone, and that social events be structured to allow the children of the union to get to know one another in a relaxed setting.

Chapter 45

1. g, f, a, b, e, d, c

2. c

3. a

4. a

5. b

6. b

7. b

8. a

9. b

10. d, e, c, b, a

11. a

12. a

13. b, a, c

14. c

15. c

16. b

17. The couple is experiencing an actual loss of an external object, in this case the family pet, which has led to a grief response. Because each person experiences loss differently and progresses through the grief process differently, the nurse should assess each individual's response to the loss. The nurse needs to be aware of the signs and symptoms of dysfunctional grief, which include alterations in relationships with others, hostility toward others (in this case, anger against the pet who is still alive), extreme guilt (which the husband may be experiencing because he was out of town when the pet died), change in activity levels, feelings of worthlessness, and depression. The nurse can encourage the couple to talk to each other about their feelings, verbalize and share their feelings of grief with their friends, resume usual activities like walking the surviving dog, and accept the loss as part of the natural life process. This is an elderly couple, so the nurse needs to be sensitive to developmental factors of aging that may be affected by loss and grief.

18. The client is experiencing situational loss, loss of income (financial independence), and loss of self-esteem, self-worth, and social status. Nursing diagnosis: *Altered Family Processes: dysfunctional grieving and powerlessness.* Interventions include nursing assessment for signs of depression or potential self harm, encouraging the client to talk with his family members,

and a referral to a support group and job counseling.

Chapter 46

1. b, e, d, f, g, h, c, a

2. b

3. c

4. anhedonia

5. a

6. d

7. a

8. b

9. c

10. a

11. b

12. c

13. The patient needs a gynecological examination, which should include clinical breast examination, mammogram, and a Pap smear. It is likely that the client is menopausal since her last menstrual period was over a year ago. The patient needs to be educated regarding health promotion activities to prevent diseases associated with the aging process. She needs to be educated about body changes associated with menopause. The nurse can recommend the client use a water-soluble lubricant during sexual intercourse, which will increase vaginal lubrication and make sexual intercourse more comfortable.

14. PLISSIT is an intervention strategy used by a health professional working with clients diagnosed with sexual

dysfunction or altered sexuality patterns that guides the practitioner from a low level of intervention to the most intensive level. The acronym stands for:

P = permission. The nurse through interacting in a professional manner, providing privacy, and asking open-ended questions gives the client permission to talk about sexual issues.

LI = limited information. The nurse shares some information about sexual issues and the client's diagnosis; for instance, the nurse may state, "It is common for people with chronic pain to wonder how they can continue to express their sexual needs without experiencing pain."

SS = specific suggestions. The nurse can provide the client with information that will help resolve the problem;, for instance, for a patient in chronic pain the nurse can suggest that the couple engage in other types of sexually gratifying expressions besides intercourse, like cuddling and massage.

IT = intensive therapy. When low level interventions are not successful, the client should be referred to a certified sex therapist.

Chapter 47

1. a, c, g, d, h, e, f, b

2. b

3. psychoneuroimmunology

4. a

5. d

6. b

7. d

8. c

9. f, a, e, g, d, h, c, b

10. c, d, a, b

11. b

12. b

13. a

14. b

15. a

16. b, c, e, d, a

17. d

18. d

19. b

20. This nurse is experiencing the third phase of burnout: continuous deterioration. He is experiencing physiological symptoms, and if he doesn't adapt and make some changes a crisis may develop. First, his state of health should be his first priority. The headaches and insomnia should be evaluated by a health professional in order to assess the etiology of these symptoms. Second, the nurse should adopt stress-reducing behaviors, particularly exercise, healthful eating, and progressive relaxation or meditation. Third, the nurse should speak with his manager to explore how staffing shortages can be best handled. A solution to the shortage must be developed, one that does not solely rely on current staff filling in staffing gaps. The nurse must also learn to say no and not feel guilt-ridden when he declines overtime. Finally, the nurse must recognize his personal response to stress and adopt coping mechanisms to prevent illness.

Chapter 48

1. c

2. d

3. b

4. e

5. c

6. b

7. e, d, b, c, a

8. b

9. Jehovah's Witnesses

10. c

11. d

12. remote intercessory prayer

13. individuating-reflective

14. b

15. Roman Catholics believe that Communion is Christ's body and blood, and that by receiving the host, one is nourished spiritually and brought closer to God. The nurse may ask the priest to administer a very small piece of the unleavened host, as it will be dissolved by salivary amylase and absorbed without entering the gastrointestinal system. The nurse should ask that her client not drink the wine, as this is not appropriate for a client who is NPO. The client who receives the host and foregoes the wine receives the same spiritual graces as one who partakes of both.